NEURODEGENERATIVE DISEASES - LABORATORY AND CLINICAL RESEARCH

AMYOTROPHIC LATERAL SCLEROSIS

SYMPTOMS, TREATMENT AND PROGNOSIS

NEURODEGENERATIVE DISEASES - LABORATORY AND CLINICAL RESEARCH

Additional books in this series can be found on Nova's website under the Series tab.

Additional E-books in this series can be found on Nova's website under the e-book tab.

NEUROSCIENCE RESEARCH PROGRESS

Additional books in this series can be found on Nova's website under the Series tab.

Additional E-books in this series can be found on Nova's website under the e-book tab.

NEURODEGENERATIVE DISEASES - LABORATORY AND CLINICAL RESEARCH

AMYOTROPHIC LATERAL SCLEROSIS

SYMPTOMS, TREATMENT AND PROGNOSIS

KATASHI SEGAWA
AND
RYOTA IJICHI
EDITORS

NOVA BIOMEDICAL
New York

For permission to use material from this book please contact us:
Telephone 631-231-7269; Fax 631-231-8175
Web Site: http://www.novapublishers.com

LIBRARY OF CONGRESS CATALOGING-IN-PUBLICATION DATA

ISBN: 978-1-62257-679-1

Library of Congress Control Number: 2012944805

Published by Nova Science Publishers, Inc. † New York

Contents

Preface

Amyotrophic Lateral Sclerosis (ALS) or Lou Gehrig's disease is an adult-onset fatal neurodegenerative disease characterized by progressive apoptosis of upper and lower motor neurons in the brain, brainstem and spinal cord. This results in paralysis of bulbar, limb, thoracic and abdominal skeletal muscles, and death within 2-5 years of diagnosis. In this book, the authors present current research on the symptoms, treatment and prognosis of ALS. Topics include audiological profiles and hearing loss in ALS patients; the role of the lipid transcription factor and sterol regulatory element binding protein 1 (SREBP1) in ALS; molecular targeted therapy for ALS; physical and communication disabilities in ALS; psychological interventions for ALS patients and their caregivers; and a study of ALS progression and propagation.

Chapter 1 – Although it is well-known that amyotrophic lateral sclerosis (ALS) primarily affects motor neurons, the involvement of sensory pathways in the disease is currently receiving more attention. There is a dearth of information regarding the atypical effects of ALS, resulting in limited understanding of the vulnerability of for example the auditory system.

The presence of hearing loss negatively impacts on participation across all communicative contexts, stripping individuals of autonomy and self-worth, ultimately resulting in withdrawal and isolation. These factors form the foundation of individual desire to pursue life-prolonging measures. Hearing loss, combined with dysarthria and the use of augmentative and alternative communicative strategies, implies that individuals with ALS require additional support to meet their daily communicative needs.

This descriptive, exploratory study aimed to describe the audiological profile of individuals with ALS. In addition, perceptions of individuals with ALS and their caregivers of the implications of auditory impairment and value of auditory diagnosis were explored.

An evaluation of auditory function was performed on eight individuals with a neurologist confirmed diagnosis of ALS. Auditory function was assessed using a comprehensive audiological test battery that included both objective and subjective measures. Perceptions related to auditory impairment were determined using the Hearing Handicap Inventory for Adults and the Hearing Experience Questionnaire.

The results of the study indicate that a high frequency sensorineural hearing loss was identified in six of the participants. Auditory handicap, as measured by the Hearing Handicap Inventory for Adults, was reported by four of the participants. Interestingly, the caregivers related more to the threats of auditory impairment and value of auditory diagnosis than individuals with ALS.

The nature of hearing loss identified in this study mimics the pattern of a presbycutic hearing loss. Participants' limited understanding of the devastating consequences of hearing loss on quality of life highlights the need for the inclusion of an audiologist as part of the multidisciplinary management team. Audiological assessment, management, counseling and education will serve to guide the process of sensory regulation and limit psychosocial threats posed by hearing loss in individuals with ALS. This will in turn promote enhanced quality of life and maintenance of individual autonomy.

Chapter 2 – Amyotrophic Lateral Sclerosis (ALS) is a progressive neurodegenerative disease which leads to disability and death. A number of potential mechanisms for the development of ALS have been proposed. Emerging evidence strongly suggests a connection between lipid metabolism abnormalities and ALS. Glutamate excitotoxicity has been also identified as one of the major contributing factors mediating cell death in ALS. The authors have recently established a causative link between glutamate excitotoxicity-induced lipid transcription factor sterol regulatory element binding protein-1 (SREBP1) activation and neuronal apoptosis in ischemic stroke. The inhibition of neuronal SREBP1 by high exogenous cholesterol or a TAT-fused short peptide (Indip) significantly protected neurons both in vitro and in vivo. More recently, the authors detected a high level of SREBP1 activation in the spinal cord tissues of the G93A mouse model of ALS and post-mortem ALS patients indicating a pivotal role for the lipid transcription factor in the pathogenesis of ALS. In this chapter, the authors will discuss their findings on NMDA subtype glutamate receptor overexcitation induced SREBP1 activation and neuronal apoptosis as well as potential therapeutic benefits of modulating this lipid transcription signaling pathway in ALS treatment.

Chapter 3 – Abnormal deposition of ubiquitinated proteins is one of the key pathological features in various neurological disorders. The aggregates are composed of some "core proteins" that are unique to diseases. In amyotrophic lateral sclerosis (ALS), two major proteins have been intensively studied: one is mutant forms of superoxide dismutase 1 (SOD1) accounting for 20% of familial ALS; another is TAR DNA binding protein 43kDa (TDP-43), a central component of ubiquitinated inclusions of sporadic ALS patients. These proteins cause diverse pathogenic cascades both intra- and extra-cellular milieu, leading to motor neuron degeneration in ALS. In particular, recent lines of evidence imply that ALS-linked misfolded proteins could serve as seeds to nucleate their native forms, and even could be propagated from cell to cell. This scenario is attracting increasing attention as a potential mechanisms underlying irreversible disease progression. Therefore, a molecular targeting against such proteins both inside and outside motor neurons is a reasonable and practical approach for ALS. Target candidates vary in size from larger species such as oligomers, protofibrils, or aggregates, to specific amino acid residues of the protein. Accordingly, one of the aims of the molecular targeting is to trap or clear aberrantly assembled proteins. Another strategy is to attack pathogenic structures localized in disease-causal proteins to prevent further misfolding. The antibody medicine perfectly fits this end due to an advantage of the target-specific recognition. Either active or passive immunization against mutant SOD1 effectively expands the longevity of ALS model mice. Moreover, several murine monoclonal antibodies recognizing only misfolded SOD1 proteins, but not native forms, have been developed, and provided a therapeutic benefit on the mutant SOD1 transgenic mice.

Furthermore, the recent advance in technology of antibody engineering allows us to transform monoclonal antibody of mouse-origin to humanized immunoglobulin or to generate a single chain of the fragment of variance (scFv) to be used for the intrabody. In addition, several small compounds are shown to prevent aggregation of mutant SOD1 or TDP-43, and high-throughput screening of more effective molecules is underway. To expand the potential of molecular targeted therapy, the structural analysis is expected for the identification of their pathogenic microdomains of ALS-linked proteins such as mutant SOD1 and TDP-43.

Chapter 4 – *Background*: The physical and communication disabilities resulting from the onset of amyotrophic lateral sclerosis (ALS) impinge on individuals' ability to remain functionally independent. This decrease in independence inevitably leads to continuously changing roles and responsibilities within the marital relationship. One of the most constructive ways in dealing with the emotions elicited by these changes is communication.

Method: This correlational study aimed to explore the relationship between the deteriorating speech of persons with ALS and the couple's perception of marital communication. Fourteen couples participated in this study. Data were collected at three-monthly intervals over a 12-month period through the administration of objective and subjective measures.

Results: The results of the study confirmed the inevitable decline in speech intelligibility across the disease progression. However, despite this decline, the relationship between the deteriorating speech and the couples' perception of marital communication was not statistically significant.

Conclusions: The assumption that communication between couples will invariably deteriorate as a result of gradually decreasing speech intelligibility is not necessarily valid. This highlights the vital importance of effective marital communication. The use of effective augmentative and alternative communication strategies has been proven to preserve the ability to develop and maintain intimate, rewarding relationships despite the presence of profound physical disabilities.

Chapter 5 – There are many psychological issues relevant to Amyotrophic Lateral Sclerosis. The progressive and currently un-stoppable nature of the disease may lead to a reaction that includes a depressive response, hopelessness and anxiety, in both ALS patients and caregivers. In a multidisciplinary ALS team, attention to psychological aspects can significantly improve the quality of life of patients and relatives. Psychologists may play an important role in care, from a bio-psycho-social perspective.

An initial psychological intervention may begin during the diagnosis phase, supporting the communication given by the physician, with attention to emotive and psychosocial aspects. After the diagnosis and during disease progression, patients and carers should be able to access a "safe place", a relationship with a professional where they can receive counselling, aimed at improving coping methods. Psychologists can increase the acceptance rate of devices such as wheelchairs, NIVs and communicators or, at least, promote a better awareness of their psychological significance. Specific counselling could be provided in the choice of invasive interventions, such as PEG of tracheostomy, and may be useful in the acceptance of end-of-life deliberations. Spiritual assistance, not strictly related to religious believes, can be very helpful to patients and their close relatives.

Psychological support may also be helpful for physicians, giving their burden of care. People who work with ALS patients are at a high risk of professional burnout. Psychological counselling may be an appropriate response to reduce this risk.

Chapter 6 – Amyotrophic lateral sclerosis (ALS) is a neurodegenerative disorder that affects 1 in 50,000 persons. Symptoms begin to develop between 40 and 70 years old, but can occur as young as 30 years of age. Also known as Lou Gehrig's disease, ALS patients demonstrate twitching and overall muscle weakness. Eventually, the disease spreads to other areas of the body, causing muscle atrophy marked by motor neuron degeneration in the central nervous system leading to loss of voluntary muscle control. Amyotrophic lateral sclerosis is a fatal disorder which typically leads to death within three to five years after initial onset of symptoms. Although the majority of ALS cases are sporadic, the exact cause is unknown. Furthermore, only 5-10% of all ALS cases are classified as familial. Current literature bolsters a mutation in the antioxidant enzyme, superoxide dismutase 1 (SOD1), as a possible causative agent, yet only 10% of all ALS patients have this specific genetic mutation. The SOD1 mutation reduces the ability to reduce harmful free radicals, thereby promoting lipid peroxidation and inducing higher levels of lipid peroxidation end products (i.e. acrolein, 4-hydroxy-2-nonenal, malondialdehyde). Lipid peroxidation is a multifaceted biochemical process involving the interaction of polyunsaturated fatty acids with oxygen- containing free radicals in turn generating a plethora of highly reactive electrophilic aldehydes. This article will focus on the relationship between amyotrophic lateral sclerosis and lipid peroxidation, specifically the current pharmacological treatments associated with the alteration of lipid metabolism to treat the symptoms of this debilitating disease.

Chapter 7 – Objective: The rostral-caudal distributions of lower motor neuron (LMN) in the pontomedullary, cervical and lumbosacral segments of the CNS are related to bulbar, upper limb and lower limb symptoms, respectively. Respiratory function will be linked to multiple motor neuron functions such as not only thoracic segment, but pontomedullary, cervical segment. A misfolding pathology involving mutant superoxide dismutase-1 and TDP-43 causing sporadic ALS has recently been suggested to spread from the site of disease onset to neighboring areas in a prion-like manner in animal models. The authors' aims were to clarify onset type in association with 5 year survival, the relationships between interval or sites from first symptoms to second symptoms and prognosis. The authors also examined the pattern of spread and direction of clinical LMN involvement over time from onset until the appearance of respiratory symptoms, and sites and frequency of normally preserved motor function at the appearance of respiratory symptoms.

Method: 150 patients with sporadic amyotrophic lateral sclerosis (ALS) underwent follow-up at 3 month intervals until the appearance of respiratory symptoms. Symptom appearances were determined using the revised version of the ALS Functional Rating Scale.

Result: Median survival with combined type onset (two regions simultaneously) was shorter (18 months) than with bulbar onset (26 months, p1/40.01). The interval from onset to involvement of the second region correlated significantly with survival, independent of particular combinations. Five year survival rate was 21% for lower limb onset, 18% for upper limb onset and 16% for bulbar onset. No patient with a rapid spread pattern (two regions within 3 months from onset) survived >5 years. In terms of cumulative occurrence, symptoms spread longitudinally to adjacent regions. Bulbar function remained preserved in 27%, lower limb function in 10% and upper limb function in 2.7%.

Conclusion: The data supports the contiguous anatomical propagation of LMN involvement in sporadic ALS.

In: Amyotrophic Lateral Sclerosis
Editors: Katashi Segawa and Ryota Ijichi
ISBN: 978-1-62257-679-1

Chapter 1

The Audiological Profile and Perceptions of Hearing Loss in Individuals with Amyotrophic Lateral Sclerosis

Elena Philippou and Karin Joubert
University of the Witwatersrand, Johannesburg, South Africa

Abstract

Although it is well-known that amyotrophic lateral sclerosis (ALS) primarily affects motor neurons, the involvement of sensory pathways in the disease is currently receiving more attention. There is a dearth of information regarding the atypical effects of ALS, resulting in limited understanding of the vulnerability of for example the auditory system.

The presence of hearing loss negatively impacts on participation across all communicative contexts, stripping individuals of autonomy and self-worth, ultimately resulting in withdrawal and isolation. These factors form the foundation of individual desire to pursue life-prolonging measures. Hearing loss, combined with dysarthria and the use of augmentative and alternative communicative strategies, implies that individuals with ALS require additional support to meet their daily communicative needs.

This descriptive, exploratory study aimed to describe the audiological profile of individuals with ALS. In addition, perceptions of individuals with ALS and their caregivers of the implications of auditory impairment and value of auditory diagnosis were explored.

An evaluation of auditory function was performed on eight individuals with a neurologist confirmed diagnosis of ALS. Auditory function was assessed using a comprehensive audiological test battery that included both objective and subjective measures. Perceptions related to auditory impairment were determined using the Hearing Handicap Inventory for Adults and the Hearing Experience Questionnaire.

The results of the study indicate that a high frequency sensorineural hearing loss was identified in six of the participants. Auditory handicap, as measured by the Hearing Handicap Inventory for Adults, was reported by four of the participants. Interestingly, the caregivers related more to the threats of auditory impairment and value of auditory diagnosis than individuals with ALS.

The nature of hearing loss identified in this study mimics the pattern of a presbycutic hearing loss. Participants' limited understanding of the devastating consequences of hearing loss on quality of life highlights the need for the inclusion of an audiologist as part of the multidisciplinary management team. Audiological assessment, management, counseling and education will serve to guide the process of sensory regulation and limit psychosocial threats posed by hearing loss in individuals with ALS. This will in turn promote enhanced quality of life and maintenance of individual autonomy.

Keywords: Atypical symptoms; hearing loss; perceptions; sensory regulation; socio-emotional consequences

INTRODUCTION

The quality of life in adults with progressive, neurodegenerative disorders is severely affected at multiple levels of functioning. This chapter will review current literature related to ALS, hearing loss and the interrelated implications of these. These factors will be discussed within the International Classification of Functioning, Health and Disability (ICF) framework. It further aims to provide evidence of the limited availability of literature related to suspected sensory involvements, such as hearing impairment in ALS. The importance of auditory function for maintenance of quality of life will also be highlighted. The audiological profile of individuals with ALS as well as the perceptions of individuals with ALS and their caregivers of the implications of auditory impairment and value of auditory diagnosis will be discussed.

INTERNATIONAL CLASSIFICATION OF FUNCTIONING, HEALTH AND DISABILITY

The ICF is a scientific tool introduced by the World Health Organization (WHO) in a bid to establish an international framework serving to enhance functioning of health systems (WHO, 2001). The ICF provides comparable information about the experience of health and disability, based on a biopsychosocial school of thought, where disease is no longer defined in isolation by its physical consequences (Gagne, Jennings & Southall, 2009). This framework provides a coherent view of varying health perspectives (including biological, social and individual perspectives) without making the error of converging the complex notion of disability into only one of the named components (Gagne et al., 2009).

The ICF comprises classifications according to body function and structure; activities and participation, as well as contextual classifications linked to environmental and personal factors (UNESCAP, 2004). Each classification is further subdivided into categories providing an in-depth dissection of the various components considered within this framework. The first category, body functions and structures, serves to describe the physical capabilities and physiological functions of the body in relation to a specific health condition. This may include functioning at the level of the respiratory system, sensory and/or cardiovascular structure and function to name a few examples. The second category, activities, refers to the execution of tasks by the individual such as communicating, performing self-care tasks and domestic life (e.g. grocery shopping). Participation, then relates to individuals' involvement in life situations (e.g. domestic-, community-, social- and civic life, interpersonal interactions and relationships).

The ICF is further divided into two contextual categories, namely environmental and personal factors. Environmental factors are defined as the factors that 'make up the physical, social and attitudinal environment in which people live and conduct their lives' (UNESCAP, 2004, p.1) and form the external factors of the ICF (Royal College of Speech Language Therapists [RCSLT], 2007). These may include families, labour and employment services and systems available to the individual. The products and technology available to the individual, alongside the natural environmental and human made changes that facilitate maintained psychosocial wellbeing, support and relationships additionally comprise environmental factors. These include wheelchairs for mobility, adaptive equipment for eating and home modifications to accommodate these environmental assistors (Ball, Beukelman & Pattee, 2004). Personal factors comprise those internal factors that are specific to the individual and include age, gender, education, character, as well as past and current experiences (RCSLT, 2007). Personal factors are an important indicator of individual ability to cope with diagnoses and largely influence the manner in which different individuals experience disability (RCSLT, 2007).

The ICF framework has many advantages, the foremost of which is that it allows for a description of *all* difficulties experienced by an individual. This naturally leads to an intervention approach that is family-centered and committed to applying specific solutions that allow individuals to overcome activity and/or participation restrictions for enhanced quality of life (Gagne et al., 2009). The ICF additionally allows for an integration of both medical and social aspects of disease rather than focusing in entirety on the diagnosis itself. This further ensures that goals and solutions specific to the client are formulated to alleviate individual difficulties and promote optimal participation in activities considered to be limitative by the affected individual (Gagne et al., 2009). Management approaches that are efficacious in addressing activity limitations and participation restrictions show improvements in psychological and psychosocial wellbeing (Erdman, 2009). This approach to disease management therefore is positively associated with improved quality of life for the individual as well as the primary caregiver and other support systems.

The term quality of life is widely described in the literature; however a universal definition is yet to be established. Quality of life relates to the extent to which an individual is able to pursue and realize their life goals (Mitsumoto & Del Bene, 2000), while others refer to quality of life as those factors contributing to an individual's overall happiness and harmony (McLeod & Clarke, 2007). A common thread amongst all definitions, although a slightly more limiting perspective, is that it refers to general psychological wellbeing of the individual and the requirements necessary to realize this (Hallberg, Hallberg & Kramer, 2008). Poor quality of life has been identified to be closely related to individual end-life decisions (Kubler, Winter, Ludolph, Hautzinger & Birbaumer, 2005). It is reported that individuals with lower quality of life are more likely to decline life-sustaining treatments, further emphasizing the importance of a framework that considers all dimensions of individual functioning and involvement (Goldstein, Atkins, Landau, Brown & Leigh, 2006; Kubler et al., 2005).

Amyotrophic Lateral Sclerosis

ALS is confined to the upper and lower motor neurons in the motor cortex, brainstem and spinal cord (Kuhnlein et al., 2008), but in some instances cranial nerve nuclei may also be implicated (Shaw, 2005; Snell, 2001). ALS, at a clinical and electrophysiological level, is described as a disorder purely of the motor system, with a salient pathological feature of progressive motor cell injury and death (Donaghy, 1999). However, recent studies suggest that motor neuron groups are primarily but not exclusively involved in ALS; and are variable in vulnerability to degenerative processes (Isaacs et al., 2007; Shaw, 2005).

Sensory neuropathy has long since failed to be recognized as a clinical feature of the ALS spectrum, the presence of which has remained a cause of diagnostic uncertainty (Isaacs et al., 2007). It is postulated that a wider spectrum of ALS related signs and symptoms are anticipated to become clinically apparent as a result of increased life expectancy due to medical and supportive care developments (Isaacs et al., 2007; Shaw, 2005). With no cure and a growing range of symptoms, the challenge lies in prolonging independence and optimizing patient quality of life (Ng & Khan, 2011).

Prolonging independence and optimizing quality of life is best addressed with multi-disciplinary management that encompasses the symptomatic management, but also the physical, social and environmental factors spanning the spectrum of ALS (Ng & Khan, 2011). Investigation surrounding the atypical features of ALS is therefore essential for refining the standard clinical description of the disease. Further exploration, in support of the diagnostic process, also serves in reshaping the management of individuals with ALS. This will ensure that disease features at both a primary and secondary level are accommodated (Isaacs et al., 2007).

ICF and ALS

Body Structure and Function: Symptoms of ALS

The ICF defines body functions as *'physiological functions of body systems (including psychological functions)'* (WHO & UNESCAP, 2008, p. 27), while body structures are defined as *'the anatomical parts of the body such as organs, limbs and their components'* (WHO & UNESCAP, 2008, p.27). As motor neurons gradually cease to function, muscle deterioration results in severe and extensive decline in the functional abilities of individuals with ALS (Doyle & Phillips, 2001). A loss of motor ability is primarily reported as the core symptom of ALS, with minimal report and/or documentation of the sensory effects of the disease.

This section will provide a description of the motor systems involved in ALS in line with the ICF definitions of body function and structure. This will then be followed by a discussion surrounding documented sensory involvement in ALS on a broad scale spectrum and in relation to the auditory system, highlighting the dearth of information in this domain.

Motor Symptoms

Individuals with ALS are faced with a gradual loss of function. According to the categories described in the ICF, these include decline in muscular function (mobility), respiratory function (breathing), digestive function and structure (dysphagia), voice and speech functions (dysarthria), as well as investigations into the effects of ALS on eye (vision) structure (WHO & UNESCAP, 2008).

The deterioration of physical skills such as movement, functional use of the legs and arms for gross motor movements and fingers for fine motor manipulation remain key markers of the physical threats faced by individuals with ALS (Ball et al., 2004).

Dysphagia is as a key bulbar symptom. Dysphagia, in conjunction with progressive weakness of respiratory muscles, prevents reflexive cough action to enable clearance of the aspirated food (Kuhnlein et al., 2008). This may consequently lead to aspiration pneumonia and possible death (Ekberg et al., 2002). Dysphagia is documented in 86% of individuals with ALS (Kuhnlein et al., 2008). Muscular fasciculation of the tongue is reported in 64% of individuals. Fasciculation involve the simultaneous contraction of groups of muscle fibers resulting in muscular twitching (Snell, 2001). These at the level of the oral structures further compound difficulties in swallowing at the preparatory phase of the swallow (Kuhnlein et al., 2008).

The effects of ALS on the communicative system can be devastating to the individual. The gradual deterioration of motor neuron function impacts the respiratory system in the form of respiratory muscle weakness, threatening both communicative competence and long-term survival (Ball et al., 2004). Respiratory muscle strength is necessary for fulfilling its role in the process of phonation, without which weakness in vocal intensity and strength becomes evident. As a direct consequence, a decline in speech intelligibility is well documented in the ALS population (Freed, 2000; Yorkston et al., 1999). The decline is marked by impaired muscle tone affecting power and range of voice, breathing and oral movements as well as in-coordination of musculature for speech production (Duffy, 1995). Bulbar symptoms gradually become more pronounced as the disease progresses, with 93% of individuals developing dysarthria (Leigh et al., 2003; Kuhnlein et al., 2008). Dysarthria initially presents at varying levels of severity and this gradually evolves into a total loss of expressive verbal function. A total loss of expressive verbal function is reported in 80% of individuals with ALS as motor neuron deterioration progresses and motor neurons cease to function (Leigh et al., 2003).

Traditional curative interventions are currently inappropriate in the management of ALS. This, as well as the rapidly progressive nature of this disease, emphasizes the importance of acknowledging systems that are preserved while a steady decline of bodily function occurs. It is suggested that certain motor neuron groups are less vulnerable to the pathological process of degeneration (Shaw, 2005). For example, the motor neurons in the upper brain stem nuclei, the ocular nuclei, responsible for the control of eye movements, remain functional. The reduced vulnerability of the ocular nuclei therefore allow non-verbal, expressive communicative abilities to be somewhat maintained through the use of eye gaze and -tracking. With maintained visual function, the importance of augmentative and alternative communication (AAC) strategies become central to maintaining communicative competence amidst deterioration of verbal expressive abilities (Ball et al., 2004). The reduced vulnerability of these visual motor neuron groups further support the need to determine the susceptibility of other systems, such as the auditory system, to the ALS degenerative process.

The current study thus placed emphasis on determining auditory impairment as a possible sensory symptom of ALS.

Sensory Symptoms

In recent years various studies have explored the involvement of sensory neuropathy in a disease dominated largely by motor dysfunction (Isaacs et al., 2007; Mondelli, Rossi, Passero, & Guazzi, 1993). Isaacs et al. (2007) reported that sensory symptoms were identified in 50% of participants diagnosed with ALS (*N* = 111). These symptoms were confirmed with electrophysiological investigations, confirming the high incidence of sub-clinical, progressive sensory dysfunction (Isaacs et al., 2007). The involvement of the autonomic system, basal ganglia, dorsal columns, spinocerebellar tracts and extra-motor cortex were documented in 2-10% of these individuals. Furthermore, a 30% reduction in the total number of myelinated nerve fibers was reported in participants with ALS in contrast to a control group (Isaacs et al., 2007). Earlier studies support the presence of sensory dysfunction in ALS to a lesser extent in 13-22% of participants (Mondelli et al., 1993; Theys, Peeters & Robberecht, 1999). These differences may be accounted for by the diagnostic limitations of electrophysiological investigations used in these earlier studies. A later study exploring sensory involvement in ALS revealed a larger number of individuals presenting with normal sensory functions than previously reported. In this study (*N* = 88), a total of 20 participants presented with abnormalities within sensory parameters (Pugdhal et al., 2007). The study concluded that these findings were suggestive of unaffected sensory nerve function in ALS. It was however later acknowledged by the authors of this study, that a high probability exists that sensory nerve dysfunction is a representation of a variant of the disease and hence could not be conclusively discarded based on the participants from that study alone (Pugdahl et al., 2007). It was furthermore suggested that sensory involvement may have been underestimated since electrodiagnostic tests were not included in the test protocol (Pugdahl et al., 2007).

One of the sensory symptoms infrequently documented in individuals with ALS, is hearing loss (Gourie-Devi & Suresh, 1988; Maier et al., 2009). The auditory system comprises the outer, middle and inner ear. The outer ear region comprises the pinna, the ear canal and the tympanic membrane (Musiek & Baran, 2007). The pinna collects sound and directs it into the ear canal reaching the tympanic membrane, which is set into vibratory motion. This motion is transmitted along the ossicles of the middle ear namely, the incus, malleus and the stapes (Musiek & Baran, 2007). The ossicles serve to stimulate vibratory motion from the air medium of the outer ear to the liquid medium of the inner ear stimulating the cochlea, or the organ of hearing. This vibratory motion stimulates the transmission of the sound signal along the auditory nerve to the auditory cortex of the brain translating these signals into audible sound (Musiek & Baran, 2007). Uninterrupted transmission of the sound signal from the outer ear through to the level of the auditory cortex results in normal hearing abilities. In instances where sound is not efficiently conducted through the outer and/or middle ear, a conductive hearing loss (CHL) arises. CHL can frequently be medically or surgically corrected. Damage to the auditory system at the level of the cochlea and/or auditory nerve may result in a sensorineural hearing loss (SNHL). This can be further classified to be either a cochlear or retrocochlear loss, depending on the level of the auditory pathway at which damage occurs (Musiek & Baran, 2007). Although SNHL generally cannot be reversed, rehabilitation methods and assistive devices are available to assist in achieving improved sensory regulation.

Madras Pattern of Motor Neuron Disease (MMND), a form of ALS, was reported by Gourie-Devi and Suresh (1988). Individuals with MMND present with an age of disease onset that is at least a decade earlier than typical adult-onset ALS. Bilateral SNHL and bilateral facial nerve involvement are noted to be present in these individuals. This supports indications of sensory involvement in the ALS spectrum of disease.

Audiological testing of individuals with MMND provided evidence for hearing impairment (Gourie-Devi & Suresh, 1988). Auditory testing revealed a bilateral SNHL in ten out of 11 participants, whilst one participant presented with a unilateral SNHL. The presence of sensorineural impairment suggests damage either within the region of the inner ear (cochlea) and/or along the auditory nerve (retrocochlear) leading to the auditory cortex. This study did not report site of lesion testing to further isolate the specific location of auditory impairment. Severity varied amongst participants in this study with 50% presenting with a severe loss and the remainder with a mild-moderate loss (Gourie-Devi & Suresh, 1988). While bilateral sensorineural hearing impairment remains a main feature of MMND, the presence of hearing impairment in individuals with typical adult onset ALS has yet to be conclusively reported.

A single retrospective study provided the first hint of evidence linked to auditory involvement in adult onset ALS and included reports of hyperacusis (Maier et al., 2009). The latter has yet to be reported in ALS. All three participants in this study had undergone tracheostomy (35 months, 26 months and 25 months respectively since disease onset) and received long-term ventilation. Following retrospective review of these three cases, Maier et al. (2009) reported bilateral hearing impairment for all three participants. The test battery applied to the above study included pure tone audiometry and auditory evoked potentials, while structural lesions in the middle ear were clinically and pathoanatomically excluded (Maier et al., 2009). Speech audiometry measures were not included in this test battery.

The presence of SNHL is etiologically unknown however its presentation in two of the three participants suggested the presence of a neurodegenerative process with involvement of the auditory system (Maier et al., 2009). Sensorineural hearing impairment suggests damage within the inner ear region and/or along the auditory nerve leading to the auditory cortex. The cochlear organ of the inner ear comprises two types of neurons called the Type I and Type II afferent neurons (Spoendlin, 1971; Spoendlin & Schrott, 1989). These afferent neurons or sensory receptors are activated by the inner hair cells of the organ of Corti and are responsible for the innervations of the cochlear inner hair cells. This occurs at synapses whereby glucomate neurotransmitters communicate signals to the primary auditory neurons. The dendrites of these neurons belong to the auditory nerve, later uniting with the vestibular nerve to form the eighth cranial nerve – the vestibularcochlear or auditory nerve (Marieb, 2001). The auditory nerve is responsible for carrying the sound signal to the auditory cortex of the brain, beginning at the spinal ganglia (Marieb, 2001). Type I spinal ganglion neurons are large and myelinated whilst Type II neurons are smaller and unmyelinated (Spoendlin & Schrott, 1989). Type I afferent neurons comprise 95% of the neurons exclusively connected to the inner hair cells. Type II afferent neurons comprise 5% of the spinal ganglion cells and supply the outer hair cells (Spoendlin, 1979; Spoendlin & Schrott, 1989). The findings of the study conducted by Isaacs et al. (2007) indicated a 30% reduction of myelinated fibers occurs as a sensory consequence of ALS. The presence of a high percentage of myelinated neurons along the auditory pathway suggests that the effect of a 30% decline in myelinated fibers may threaten auditory ability. This further supports the hypothesis that a hearing loss of a sensorineural nature in individuals with ALS is a viable consideration in need of more thorough exploration and research.

In contrast to SNHL is the hypothesis that paralysis of the tensor tympani muscle, as a result of bulbar palsy symptoms, could result in a CHL. The auditory system is protected from loud stimuli by the tensor tympani muscle, which pulls the malleus medially resulting in the damping of vibrations in the ossicles. This results in reduced sound amplitude (Marieb, 2001). This damping leads to in smaller amplitude of vibratory motion along the remaining components of the auditory pathway and consequently a reduction in the loudness of the sound signal (Marieb, 2001). An alternative hypothesis may be linked to the paralysis of the tensor and levator veli palatini muscles, which pose a threat to the mechanical properties of the Eustachian tube. The impaired ability to actively dilate and increase the lumen in the cross-sectional region of the Eustachian tube arises as a result of bulbar palsy symptoms (Ghadiali, Swarts & Doyle, 2003). This leads to insufficient forces being applied to the membraneous wall of the Eustachian tube during swallowing. The latter subsequently results in the development of negative middle ear pressures and places individuals at risk for developing otitis media with effusion (Ghadiali et al., 2003). The presence of otitis media would further support the hypothesis of conductive hearing impairment (Maier et al., 2009). Findings from Maier et al. (2009) support the previously undocumented presence of hearing loss in ALS as one of the possible sensory symptoms of ALS.

Sensory involvement may not be a key marker in the current ALS diagnostic process, but may rather extend the phenotype of the disease to include a clinical or subclinical axonal sensory neuropathy (Isaacs et al., 2007). It is acknowledged that the low incidence of idiopathic neuropathy in the general population may account for its occasional presentation alongside ALS (Isaacs et al., 2007). Other studies have reached parallel conclusions suggesting that sensory involvement, as part of multi-systemic degeneration is a valid claim deserving of further investigation (Pugdahl et al., 2007). Further investigation is of particular importance in light of advances in the medical management of ALS that is resulting in the extended lifespan of individuals with ALS (Isaacs et al., 2007; Pugdahl et al., 2007). This provides greater opportunities for exposing atypical symptoms, such as hearing loss, that possibly present later in the disease and threaten individual wellbeing.

Activity Limitations and Participation Restrictions: ALS

The WHO views functionality, disability and health as an interactive process (WHO & UNESCAP, 2008). In instances of impaired body structures and functions that cannot be returned to normalcy, provision of solutions to alleviate limitations at a personal and a social level become paramount to the management of the disease (WHO, 2001). It is important to view individual functioning as the interaction between an individuals' general physical health status alongside contextual factors (WHO, 2001). The ICF view activity limitations as *'difficulties in executing activities'* (WHO & UNESCAP, 2008, p. 27*)*, while participation restrictions are viewed as *'problems in involvement in life situations'* (WHO & UNESCAP, 2008, p.27*)*. This section will focus on the various activity limitations and participation restrictions faced by an individual with ALS. These will be discussed with particular emphasis on the effects on communication and more specifically the threats brought about by hearing loss.

Activities and participation include the following categories as they relate to ALS: general tasks and demands linked to mobility, self-care, interpersonal relationships, social and community life and communication. Progressive physical weakness and loss of upper and/or lower extremity function threatens individual ability to perform activities of daily living and fulfill daily demands, such as writing, dressing, driving, walking and independent management of basic hygiene (e.g. bathing, brushing teeth).

Further to this, dementia is named as a possible symptom of ALS and negatively affects an individuals' ability to perform common daily activities such as eating, bathing and continence. Restrictions in socialization and participation within group situations arise as a consequence of these limitations (UNESCAP, 2004).

Similarly, dysphagia commonly presents as a consequence of motor neuron degeneration. The difficulties in controlling liquids for fluid intake, chewing abilities and the process of deglutition further impacts daily activities and participation. It has been found that over 50% of participants with dysphagia no longer experience eating as a pleasurable activity as a direct result of the associated limitations (Ekberg et al., 2002). Dysphagia directly affects the ability to eat and drink independent of risk. This in turn threatens individual participation in all social situations centered on dining experiences (e.g. restaurants, dinner invitations). Feelings of exclusion, isolation and distress during mealtimes were reported by participants in this study consequently resulting in increased reluctance and avoidance of eating in social settings that extend beyond the privacy of the home environment and primary caregiver (Ekberg et al., 2002). This not only threatens individual wellbeing, but places strain on the maintenance of relationships.

Respiratory muscle weakness results in individuals with ALS experiencing respiratory insufficiency (Ball et al., 2004). These symptoms include disturbed sleep, fatigue, morning headaches, increased respiratory rate, as well as poor concentration and memory (Ball et al., 2004). While assisted ventilation of a non-invasive nature has been positively associated with improving patient quality of life, invasive ventilation measures (e.g. tracheostomy) have negative effects on remaining communicative ability (Van Damme & Robberecht, 2009). Such respiratory symptoms further limit individual ability to perform activities of self-care, desire to engage in community and/or social activities and threaten the maintenance of established interpersonal relationships and/or establishing new relationships (Van Damme & Robberecht, 2009).

Dysarthria is identified as one of the most debilitating deficits experienced by individuals with ALS (Leigh et al., 2003; Kuhnlein et al., 2008). The communication process relies on a two-way exchange whereby individuals receive and provide information. For this exchange to be effective, intact verbal expression and auditory reception is necessary. A breakdown in one or both of these processes, results in a breakdown in interactive exchange (Glennen & DeCoste, 1997). Dysarthria impairs verbal communicative abilities and negatively affects communicative success in activities of speech. This includes making requests, expressing concerns and/or sharing information for functional or social purposes (Aronson, Ramig, Winholtz & Silber, 1992; Kuhnlein et al., 2008). Communication is a critical component in promoting psychological independence, establishing social closeness and maintaining independence in activities of daily living. Deterioration or loss of communicative abilities increases dependence on others, strips individuals of autonomy and in time provides evidence of a decline in social and emotional wellbeing (Ball et al., 2004). Activity limitations as a result of dysarthria further include reduced speech intelligibility and communicative ability.

This has serious implications on participation and creates restrictions to an individuals' participation at a level of social functioning i.e. church gatherings, family functions, and community gatherings. Furthermore, medical autonomy i.e. expressing thoughts, concerns or requests, directly related to the management of ALS, may become restricted further damaging individual perception of control and desire to engage in the decision-making process.

A breakdown in auditory reception amongst this population would largely be brought about by deterioration or loss of auditory function. Hearing loss is often unrecognized and undertreated as a health disorder, despite the marked implications this has on individual quality of life (Dalton et al., 2002). Hearing impairment in individuals with ALS may further be exacerbated by the additional symptoms and loss of function experienced by the affected individuals.

Activity Limitations and Participation Restrictions: Hearing Loss and ALS

The prevalence of hearing impairment is reported to occur in 10 – 20 % of the population worldwide as a consequence of various auditory pathologies (Mathers, Smith & Concha, 2003). Age-related hearing loss, or presbycusis, occurs in approximately 46% of the population aged 48-65 years (Yueh, Shapiro, MacLean & Shekelle, 2003). It is important to note that the age range in which ALS diagnosis and progression occurs typically correlates with the range in which presbycutic hearing loss presents. It is therefore postulated that individuals with ALS may at some stage experience hearing impairment, regardless of whether this is directly or indirectly related to the ALS itself.

The impact of hearing loss on activities and participation in daily life does not vary according to the cause of onset, but is rather based on severity and the functional obstacles experienced (Nachtegaal et al., 2009). This provides further support for the relevance of auditory testing within this population group. The consequent findings may then be instrumental in guiding sensory regulation of auditory function, for an unobstructed process of communicative interaction.

Hearing impairment inevitably affects health-related quality of life at a psychosocial level (Chia et al., 2007). It introduces a range of activity limitations and restrictions to successful participation in daily life. Hearing loss in later adulthood may trigger an identity crisis and reactive depression may occur (Dewane, 2010). Associated psychosocial effects of hearing impairment include anxiety, distress, loneliness, somatization and poor social functioning (Nachtegaal et al., 2009). Additional consequences of impaired hearing include difficulties with localizing sounds and/or the threat of being unable to detect warning signals (Hallberg et al., 2008). The effects of hearing impairment may extend to activities such as watching television, understanding whispering, being unaware someone is talking and/or listening to the radio - all of which form important contributions to maintaining a sense of involvement in the world around. This is particularly relevant when dealing with a loss of multiple other functions (Dewane, 2010). Hearing loss furthermore introduces a false sense of understanding due to misinterpretation of speech sounds, creating feelings of disillusionment (Nachtegaal et al., 2009).

Since a sense of belonging is largely associated with mental health, a loss of hearing creates a psychological sensory confinement with harmful negative effects on individual belonging and mental wellbeing (Dewane, 2010). This has serious implications on an individuals' ability to maintain their identity, potentially resulting in communicative limitations. This leads to difficulty thinking, concentration and boredom. The resultant inattentiveness, distraction, isolation and depression leads to the most serious consequence of hearing loss - abandoning participation (Dewane, 2010; Gates & Mills, 2005).

The social stigmas associated with hearing impairment in adults include labels such as troublesomeness, slow-wittedness and tiresomeness (Dewane, 2010). The internalization of such prejudices result in a further blow to an individuals' self-esteem leading to depressive exhaustion and marked changes in individual personality (Dewane, 2010). When considering dementia and hearing loss it is also worthwhile to consider the related changes in character and personality. Where changes in character and personality occur, subjective detection of altered cognitive abilities may be impeded by the possibility of impaired hearing. This subsequently precludes conclusive decision-making and recurrent communicative breakdown continues (Leigh et al., 2003). In instances where this is a direct result of impaired hearing, damaging consequences for psychosocial wellbeing and interpersonal relationships continue to be exacerbated in the midst of blurred diagnosis (Erber & Scherer, 1999).

Restrictions on an individuals' execution of activities involving an exchange of information (e.g. expressing needs and wants, medical enquiries, legal interactions such as drafting of wills) impose barriers to independent functioning. Dysarthria in combination with hearing impairment results in voluntary or involuntary exclusion from social situations for fear of humiliation, isolation and loss of dignity (Foley et al, 2007; Kelly et al., 2003). Individuals typically report experiencing a lack of authenticity and feelings of alienation from people and activities that previously may have created a sense of belonging. This gradually leads to social exclusion. Themes including a loss of autonomy and lack of dignity that arise as a result of social exclusion are closely related to individual desire to hasten death when living with a terminal illness (Kelly et al., 2003). The effects of hearing loss can therefore not be underestimated as a secondary feature separate from the disease itself.

It has been found that female participants with hearing impairment experience feelings of annoyance, irritation and anger (Hallberg et al., 2008). Male participants, who generally failed to recognize the extent of their hearing difficulties, reported these feelings to a lesser extent. The application of non-verbal communication strategies, serving as a solution to facilitate the enhancement of participation in daily life, was also reported. However, these behaviours were noted more readily in female participants in contrast to male participants who generally showed more denial associated with hearing loss (Garstecki & Erler, 1999; Hallberg et al., 2008). The denial of hearing loss hinders success in addressing activity limitations and amplifies the restrictions on participation.

Despite the negative consequences brought about by hearing impairment, individuals with hearing impairment underestimate the consequences and the extent of withdrawal from interactions and/or avoidance of listening situations (Hallberg et al., 2008; Dalton et al., 2003). It is postulated that the avoidance of listening situations occurs as a result of the individuals' failure to accept their difficulties and pursue audiological rehabilitation (Dalton et al., 2003). It is further suggested that certain individuals show preference for self-deception as a means of reducing the discrepancies between reality and their perceived self-image (Hallberg & Barrenas, 1995). In a disease such as ALS where individuals deal with the constant need to redefine their perceived image according to the gradual loss of functional abilities, secondary impairments, such as hearing loss, may not be readily acknowledged, and are consequently addressed with less urgency, if at all.

The effects of hearing impairment on the social and psychological wellbeing of individuals are hence profound (Ross & Deverell, 2004). The resultant social withdrawal, avoidance of previously positively associated hobbies and/or activities, exclusion from social exchange and loss of empowerment pose obvious risks, further increasing the demands and stress of living with ALS. Essentially, the absence of communicative success results in the patient becoming locked in; physically present, although immobile; and cognitively aware, amidst social exclusion (Ross & Deverell, 2004).

Contextual Factors: ALS and Hearing Loss

The contextual factors outlined by the ICF framework comprise external environmental factors and internal personal factors (WHO, 2001). Environmental factors that have an impact on the functioning of individuals with disability include the products and technology available to the individual. Alongside this are the natural environmental and human made changes that serve to facilitate psychosocial wellbeing, support and relationships. Personal factors such as individual attitudes and coping mechanisms for acknowledging and accepting diagnosis, alongside environmental factors are integral to the maintenance of individual quality of life extending beyond the physical definition of the disease (WHO, 2001). For an individual with ALS, emphasis needs to be directed at maintaining and improving quality of life (McLeod & Clarke, 2007). Factors within the environment can hence be instrumental in either facilitating or limiting activities or participation restrictions faced by individuals with ALS.

Individual attitudes and the attitudes of those around them form a key component in dealing with disease. The diagnosis of ALS evokes various strong psychological reactions to the constant adjustments to the loss of functional abilities, loss of autonomy and self and the reality of death as the disease progresses (Averill, Kasarskis & Segerstrom, 2007). These experiences of loss arouse signs of depression, including withdrawal and self-isolation, often resulting in a decline in individual willingness to prolong and sustain life (Erdman, 2009; Kelly et al., 2003). Beck's cognitive theory of depression suggests that the cognitive profile of depression is set off and revolves around themes of loss (Erdman, 2009). The ICF framework supports the notion that promoting quality of life extends beyond the alleviation of physical burden and is rather more closely correlated to suffering, social support and sense of autonomy (McLeod & Clarke, 2007). This is supported by Simmons, Bremer, Robbins, Walsh and Fisher (2000) who found that the compensation for physical symptoms in ALS does not markedly correlate to the alleviation of emotional distress. The latter is however more closely related to the existential and psychological aspects of life.

In a study conducted to understand the personal perceptions of quality of life of individuals living with a progressive disease, participants expressed a strong desire to maintain their sense of self and to be viewed independently from their disability (Foley et al., 2007). It was further found that the ability of an individual to maintain a level of independence is largely determined by the interactions he/she engages in (Foley et al., 2007). This emphasizes the importance of functional auditory ability, without which these interactive processes are jeopardized.

Dignity was raised as an important theme linked to the individuals' need to be respected and viewed independently of the disability. The lack of this was closely related to individual desires to hasten death (Foley et al., 2007; Kelly et al., 2003). Control, in terms of individual need to be *in* control and acknowledgement of the uncertainty paired with ALS, creates feelings of vulnerability and dependency. Control is also linked to the sharing of thoughts and being respected in the decision-making process, which additionally add to the psychological effects of ALS (Foley et al., 2007).

Studies have indicated that individuals with progressive neurological diseases inevitably adapt to the disease and the progressive loss of physical function through a process of acknowledgement (Hardiman et al., 2004; Ross & Deverell, 2004). These individuals acknowledge the challenge of coping with feelings of loss and the strain of being physically dependent on others. This, when paired with feelings of vulnerability, results in a shift of focus being placed on maintaining the locus of control at an interactive level, thereby empowering themselves as autonomous in daily interactive experiences (Foley et al., 2007; Hallberg, 1999). Essentially, individuals are able to lower their personal expectations surrounding physical activity levels. They redirect this attention to other aspects of their lives in order to maintain a sense of self-worth and view themselves as purposeful contributors to the world around them (Hallberg et al., 2008; Ng & Khan, 2011). It is therefore through the control of environmental factors (such as the alleviation of certain symptoms, support and individual attitudes) that individual participation is maintained.

It is postulated that the obstacles to effective communication faced by individuals with ALS may be brought about by dysarthria, hearing loss or a combination of the two. This threatens autonomy and engagement in activities of daily living. Individual attitude towards ALS, living with the various physical effects and the associated emotional and social consequences plays a critical role in the manner an individual deals with ALS (Ball et al., 2004). The use of products and technology such as wheelchairs to aid mobility, adaptive eating equipment to accommodate eating difficulties and changes to the environment such as ramps and home modifications to accommodate the changes in mobility can promote an improved attitude towards life (Ball et al., 2004).

Similarly, environmental factors related to communication difficulties (e.g. speech and hearing) can also enhance quality of life for individuals with ALS. Various communication-based strategies have been developed to facilitate the communicative success of individuals with dysarthria and subsequently reduce the activity limitations they face (Kuhnlein et al., 2008; Murphy, 2004; Leigh et al., 2003; Grauman, Betke, Gips & Bradski, 2001; Lasker & Bedrosian, 2000). AAC strategies assist where deterioration in hand function and functional speech prevents alternate forms of communication (Leigh et al., 2003; Lasker & Bedrosian, 2000). These may include unaided strategies (such as facial expressions, gestural communication and eye movement) or low technology systems (such as alphabet cues and boards, and communication boards). Often eye gaze, a form of direct selection where individuals perform pre-learned eye movements directed to a communication board, may be utilized (Grauman et al., 2001). High technology AAC systems (such as speech generation systems or specialized eye tracking technology) may also be used to facilitate expressive communicative abilities (Murphy, 2004).

The use of AAC strategies and aids accommodate loss of expressive language abilities in ALS, however facilitation of auditory deficits amongst this population is not met with equal urgency and importance (Dalton et al., 2003). This occurs despite the extent to which psychological and psychosocial factors related to hearing impairment restrict participation in daily activities (Gates & Mills, 2005). Solutions to auditory reception breakdown should consequently not be excluded from the management of individuals with ALS.

The benefits of achieving sensory regulation, often through the introduction of a hearing amplification device (e.g. a hearing aid) or communication training, positively contribute to quality of life. It has been found that the use of hearing aids demonstrate positive effects on an individuals' self-perceived hearing handicap, further supporting the benefit of identifying impairment and promoting the urgency for achieving successful sensory regulation (Tesch-Romer, 1997). Communication training, offered by audiologists, offers paired communication partner strategies to alleviate the extent of communicative breakdown. These strategies include non-verbal communication training (such as lip reading or sitting closer to a speaker), environmental modifications (furniture rearrangement, lighting changes) and psychosocial support (counseling) (Hallberg et al., 2008; Kramer, 2008; Michaud, Burnand & Stiefel, 2004). These rehabilitative approaches serve to enhance communicative effectiveness and in doing so promote social inclusion (Gates & Mills, 2005; Michaud et al., 2004).

These rehabilitation or facilitation-based solutions form the foundation of the ICF framework, and serve to implement solutions that will overcome, alleviate or minimize difficulties. This is particularly relevant in instances where disease is chronic and bodily structural and/or functional damage cannot be returned to normalcy (Gagne et al., 2009). Equipping the individual with the skills to communicate, assists in keeping him actively involved in the world around and lends the individual a degree of independence and autonomy in the face of irreversible physical decline and loss of physical function.

In addition to the personal effects of hearing impairment, hearing loss also threatens the functional success of relationships within the family structure (Hallam, Ashton, Sherbourne & Gailey, 2008). The value of support systems is highlighted by the ICF as an environmental factor contributing to the overall wellbeing of the individual (WHO, 2001). Numerous studies have reported that hearing loss does place considerable strain on family structures and enhance their vulnerability to failure (Hallam et al., 2008; Armero, 2001). However, the effects on the family/support structure appear to vary based on the extent and severity of the hearing loss. Family members of individuals with hearing impairment report significant increase in frustration and irritation and the effects are documented to reverberate throughout the family system (Dewane, 2010; Armero, 2001). The negative impact hearing impairment poses on intimate relationships, emphasizes the maladaptive behaviour and coping strategies implemented by a couple in crisis due to hearing impairment (Armero, 2001). Caregivers of hearing impaired individuals identified emotional consequences including deep resentment, anger, reclusiveness and depression. The caregivers were reported to be twice more likely to complain about reduced social activities than the individuals with hearing impairment. Affected individuals in turn begin to experience isolation from immediate family structures and a sense of guilt for their role in the breakdown of successful communication (Armero, 2001). This is supported by Dewane (2010) who reported that individuals with hearing impairment experience feelings of remorse for the constant need to request repetition. They further reported distrust, nervousness, irritability and reduced self-image associated with the effects of hearing loss on a family structure.

The devastating effects of hearing impairment threaten the maintenance of caregiver-patient relationships and family structures. This is particularly true when hearing impairment is superimposed on the additional challenges faced by individuals with ALS and their families. The effects of hearing loss increase the psychological burden posed on individual perspectives of autonomy and quality of life, in addition to having a marked impact on caregiver dynamics.

The process of providing an individual with the options available to alleviate or minimize the effects of a hearing impairment, allows for an inclusive management approach where the individual is able to prioritize rehabilitation goals. This promotes the likelihood of individual motivation to apply the outlined strategies, which have shown to have a positive effect on individual attitudes and behaviours as they encourage a sense of autonomy, empowerment and personal growth (Gagne et al., 2009). This in turn will promote positive dynamics within an individuals' support system.

The ICF framework therefore views the individual holistically and promotes enhanced activity and participation in daily living, through manipulating environmental factors to limit the extent of the physical, social and emotional effects of ALS. To achieve success, a multi-disciplinary approach to patient management is paramount.

Multi-Disciplinary Management in ALS

The management of progressive degenerative diseases should be directed towards managing the primary presenting symptoms and rehabilitating secondary symptoms (either directly or indirectly related to the disease itself). It is the role of the multi-disciplinary team (MDT) to manage all symptoms in a manner that affords the individual the time and ability to dissociate worth from physical capability and reassign value to autonomy and maintenance of dignity at a psychological, social and existential level (Foley et al., 2007). The primary members of the ALS management team include the neurologist, respiratory physician and gastroenterologist. These team members are responsible for the management of physical symptoms associated with breathing and swallowing, without which prolonged survival would not be possible. The secondary members of the ALS MDT team are typically reported to comprise of the care coordinator, caregiver, general practitioner, occupational therapist, physiotherapist, speech therapist, dietician, social worker, palliative care teams and psychologist (Leigh et al., 2003; Mitsumoto & Del Bene, 2000). Although hearing impairment has been identified as one of the significant risk factors associated with a reduced quality of life (Hallberg et al., 2008), the audiologist is not included in the MDT for individuals diagnosed with ALS. This highlights an important gap in the process of promoting and enhancing quality of life amongst the target population. Allowing an untrained professional to deal with the effects of hearing loss may result in an underestimation of the extent of frustration or misattribution the level of frustration (Dewane, 2010). The misattribution of the changes in personality associated with hearing impairment lead to unintentional mismanagement of the patient, further exacerbating the consequences of hearing loss (Dewane, 2010).

Ward, Phillips, Smith and Moran (2003) highlighted the importance of multi-disciplinary teamwork in patient management as an essential cornerstone to effectively managing individual needs and wants. An evaluation of the benefits of attending clinics catering specifically to the needs of individuals with ALS revealed that clinic attendance was associated with a 47.3% decrease in one-year mortality risk (Traynor et al., 2003). A 7.5 month extension for median survival was documented, while an extended 9.6 month prognostic improvement was documented for individuals with bulbar onset ALS. This positive prognostic data was attributed to be a result of individuals being exposed to the coordinated symptomatic and disease-modifying therapies and treatments available as well as a consistent support structure (Traynor et al., 2003). Coordinated services are believed to eliminate the disjointed, overwhelming plethora of support services available to individuals with ALS and their families (Ward et al., 2003). In contrast, the use of fragmented services and referrals result in delays in referral time frames, follow up and inter-professional communication, inevitably leading to misguided decision-making (Ward et al., 2003).

While the outcomes of coordinated services support the benefits of a multi-disciplinary approach to individual management, social, emotional and economic factors also play a role in attending such clinics (Ward et al., 2003). The implications of hearing impairment on social and emotional wellbeing, threaten individual willingness and motivation to attend such clinics, further bringing to light the value and relevance of inclusion of the auditory discipline within the ALS management team.

Conclusion

ALS is now referred to as a multi-system disease (Shaw, 2005; Isaacs et al., 2007; Pugdahl et al., 2007). The likelihood of ALS-related sensory degeneration, such as hearing loss, is suggested as a possible presentation of disease variants. The use of invasive ventilation promotes the prolongation of disease course allowing neuronal categories that are susceptible to degeneration to become clinically apparent (Isaacs et al., 2007; Shaw, 2005). Furthermore, the use of long-term ventilation as a life prolonging measures increases the clinical relevance of diagnosing atypical symptoms such as hearing loss (Maier et al., 2009). This is especially relevant in the older age groups where the associated natural decline in hearing ability is prevalent. The importance of clinically relevant research related to the wider spectrum of ALS-associated features is essential and will assist in designing appropriate management plans for the individuals diagnosed with ALS. This is critically important for the purpose of complex decision making as well as the modification of electronic communication systems and palliative care (Maier et al., 2009). Despite the tangential shifts from health-related symptoms to the social effects of a disease, as supported by the ICF, the effects of ALS related to aspects of daily survival are often not viewed to be directly disease-related and hence are less readily addressed (Hardiman et al., 2004). The secondary symptoms that arise as a direct or indirect result of ALS are likely to significantly impact on quality of life and threaten participation in activities of daily living. Failing to acknowledge these symptoms ultimately impacts individual ability to take control of the disease and in contrast allows the disease to control the individual (Hardiman et al., 2004). Acknowledging the presence of hearing loss therefore ensures necessary modifications to facilitate receptive communication abilities. This in turn facilitates communicative success and promotes individual participation in daily living to proceed in a manner that is conducive to the maintenance of social inclusion and autonomy.

Due to the dearth of information on the effects of sensory degeneration in ALS on the auditory system, the question of whether individuals with ALS present with hearing loss was posed.

Methodology

Aims

The aim of the study was to obtain an audiological profile of individuals with adult onset ALS. In addition, perceptions of individuals with ALS and their caregivers of the implications of auditory impairment and value of auditory diagnosis were explored.

Research Design

An exploratory, descriptive research design was employed for the purposes of the study.

Participant Selection and Description

Participant Selection

A non-probability, purposive sampling strategy was used to select participants who were representative of the ALS population in South Africa. To account for the threats of bias common to purposive sampling strategies, participants were recruited from multiple sources at a level of private and government healthcare institutions. ALS incidence and prevalence in South Africa is suggested to be consistent with worldwide figures of 1.2 per 100,000 and 5.2 per 100,000 respectively (Wijesekera & Leigh, 2007; Logroscino et al., 2008). This suggests that 66 new cases of ALS will be diagnosed in South Africa annually. At the time of this study, 158 patients were registered with the Motor Neuron Disease Association of South Africa (MNDSA), 65 of who lived in the Gauteng region where the study was conducted. A total of 44 information packs were distributed through the MNDSA, at support group meetings, an ALS online forum, private neurologists and the out-patient clinic at a local government hospital.

Participant Description

A total of 16 individuals participated in this study (See Table 1). The eight individuals with ALS, four males and four females, met the following inclusion criteria: (i) Neurologist confirmed diagnosis of ALS; (ii) Stage I – IV according to the MND Classification (Riviere et al, 1998); (iii) Between the ages of 30 and 66 years; and (iv) Proficient in English. Individuals that presented with a known hearing impairment prior to the diagnosis of ALS were excluded from the study. They were further excluded if they presented with any co-morbid factors linked closely to hearing loss, such as diabetes, excessive noise-exposure and treatment with ototoxic medication (e.g. used for cancer treatment).

The ages of participants with ALS ranged from 49.6 to 65.6 years with an average of 58.6 years (standard deviation [SD] = 4.7 years). The average time since onset of symptoms until data collection was 44.5 months (range: 16-70 months; SD = 19.87 months). The average time since diagnosis until data collection was 30.7 months (range: 18-55 months; SD =14.97 months). Of these participants, five presented with mixed onset ALS, two with spinal onset ALS and one with bulbar onset ALS. Two of the participants were in stage I of the disease progression, three in stage II and three in stage III. Only two of the participants reported that they are currently experiencing some form of hearing impairment. In addition, the eight primary caregivers of the individuals with ALS, four males and four females, were involved in the questionnaire component of the study. In addition, the eight primary caregivers of the individuals with ALS, three males and five females, were involved in the questionnaire component of the study. The average age for caregivers was 58.8 years (range: 52.2 – 66.5; SD = 2.3 years). The limited number of individuals living with ALS in South Africa, the attrition of potential participants and geographical location impacted significantly on the sample size of this study.

Table 1. Participant Description

	P1	P2	P3	P4	P5	P6	P7	P8
Individuals with ALS								
Gender	Male	Female	Male	Female	Female	Male	Female	Male
Age (in years)	65.6	49.6	61.2	58.6	59.2	62.8	57.3	57.3
Type of ALS	Mixed	Mixed	Bulbar	Spinal	Mixed	Spinal	Mixed	Mixed
MND Classification	III	II	III	II	III	I	II	I
Acknowledged auditory difficulty	No	No	No	No	Yes	No	Yes	No
Caregivers								
Gender	Female	Male	Female	Male	Female	Female	Male	Female
Age (in years)	59.4	44.6	59.8	66.5	52.2	61.8	59.11	56.10

Measuring Instruments and Equipment

In addition to a comprehensive audiological test battery, two questionnaires were used in the study, namely the self-developed Hearing Experience Questionnaire (HEQ) and the Hearing Handicap Inventory for Adults (HHIA) (Newman, Weinstein, Jacobson, & Hug, 1990).

Audiological Test Battery

This comprehensive audiological test battery incorporated both behavioural and electrophysiological test measures to assess the different levels of auditory function. As some of the measures are reliant on either motor strength for push-button responses or individuals' ability to repeat verbally presented words, modifications were made to the specific response-mode procedures to accommodate individual participant needs and abilities. The audiological test battery included the following measures:

Case History Questionnaire

A 24-item case history questionnaire was completed by participants or their caregivers if participants were unable to hold and manage a pen due to muscle weakness or paralysis. The questionnaire comprised four categories namely personal details, auditory- and medical history and communication abilities.

Otoscopic Examination

An otoscopic examination was performed (using an otoscope) to evaluate the state of the outer ear and tympanic membrane for abnormalities and/or infection (Rappaport & Provencal, 2002).

Immitance Audiometry

This included two measures namely tympanometry and acoustic reflexes. Tympanometry evaluates middle ear status through the depiction of tympanic membrane motility as a function of variations in air pressure (Clark, Roeser & Mendrygal, 2007). Acoustic reflex testing is a measure of stapedius muscle contraction as a response to intense sound stimulation. This is performed through ipsilateral and contralateral neural pathways, thereby assisting in the differential diagnosis of middle ear-, cochlear-, retrocochlear pathologies as well as brainstem lesions (Block & Wiley, 1994).

Distortion-Product Otoacoustic Emissions (DPOAE)

This objective measure is a recording of sounds generated within the cochlea (Prieve & Fitzgerald, 2002). DPOAEs allow for information pertaining to the integrity of the cochlea to be obtained, therefore contributing to the differential diagnosis linked to auditory functioning at this level of the auditory system (Prieve & Fitzgerald, 2002).

Pure Tone Audiometry

Pure tone audiometry (air- and bone conduction) assesses hearing sensitivity as a function of frequency (Bess & Humes, 2008). Air conduction audiometry provides insight into the integrity of the auditory system as well as information relating to the symmetry, laterality, degree and configuration of individuals' hearing thresholds (Harrell, 2002). Bone conduction audiometry allows for specified information pertaining to the type of hearing loss (e.g. conductive, sensorineural or mixed) and facilitates the making of a differential diagnosis through distinguishing between outer-, middle- or inner ear pathology (Dirks, 1994).

Speech Audiometry

The most important measurable component of human auditory function must be related back to an individuals' ability to understand speech (Bess & Humes, 2008). This ability forms the foundation to participating in the majority of activities of daily living. Four speech audiometry measures were included in the test battery. The first measure, speech reception thresholds (SRT), evaluates an individuals' ability to detect and understand speech sounds at the lowest level possible (Bess & Humes, 2008). This test confirms the reliability of pure-tone audiometry results (Brandy, 2001). The second measure, most comfortable loudness (MCL) level determines a level of speech listening, which affords the patient a comfortable listening experience with an effortless ability to understand speech sounds (Brandy, 2001).

Threshold of discomfort (TD), the third speech audiometry measure, forms part of the calculation of the patients' dynamic range. Dynamic range proves useful in the differential diagnosis of cochlear versus retro-cochlear pathology (Gelfand, 2009). The last measure, speech discrimination, evaluates an individuals' ability to distinguish between sounds and recognize speech (Brandy, 2001). Speech discrimination scores guide the process of differential diagnosis associated with the possible site of pathology i.e. outer- or middle ear; cochlear or retro-cochlear.

Neurodiagnostic Auditory Brainstem Response (ABR)

This highly specific, specialized measure is capable of yielding unique diagnostic information in the differentiation of cochlear versus eigth cranial nerve pathology (Musiek, Borenstain, Hall & Schwaber, 1994). Interpretation of ABR waveforms offer insight into the latency responses at a higher level along the auditory pathway, than that which behavioural test measures are capable of (Musiek et al., 1994). ABRs have detected waveform changes in progressive degenerative diseases such as multiple sclerosis (Musiek et al., 1994). The application of this test was therefore useful in indicating the possible presence of auditory tract involvement in ALS.

Questionnaires

Hearing Experience Questionnaire (HEQ)

This self-developed questionnaire comprised 13 open-ended questions in two categories. The first category, contact with the discipline of speech pathology and audiology, served to establish whether individuals were in contact with either of the disciplines as part of their management plan. The second category, communication and hearing, directed greater focus towards participant and caregiver perceptions associated with auditory ability, functional priorities and perceived impact of hearing impairment on quality of life. The three caregiver-directed questions mirrored those of the participant-directed questions in order to draw determine variations of perceptions between the participants with ALS and their respective caregivers.

Hearing Handicap Inventory for Adults (HHIA)

The HHIA is a 25-item self-assessment checklist comprising two subscales evaluating social (12 items) and emotional (13 items) implications of hearing impairment (Newman et al., 1990). Participants were presented with three scored response options: yes (4), sometimes (2) or no (0). A total score of 100 can be obtained. Scores are calculated accordingly to reveal a 'significant handicap', 'mild-moderate handicap' or 'no handicap', while simultaneously providing insight into the nature of the handicap – be it on a social or an emotional level (Newman et al., 1990).

Data Collection Procedures

Ethical Considerations

Various ethical considerations were implemented throughout the study. The researcher obtained ethical clearance from the Human Research Ethics Committee (Medical) of the

University of the Witwatersrand before the research was conducted. Written informed consent was obtained from the MNDSA and all participants, using established and approved methods. All participants in the study were fully informed of the nature of the study and were assured of confidentiality. Each participant was required to sign a consent form, proof of his/her willingness to participate in the study and had the right to withdraw from the study at any time, without suffering any negative consequences.

Pilot Study

Once written permission was obtained from the MNDSA, two participants whom gave informed consent were included in the pilot study. These individuals were both members of the MNDSA and met the selection criteria as outlined for the main study. Both individuals were diagnosed with mixed onset ALS and were classified as 'severe' (Stage III) according the MND Classification (Riviere et al., 1998). Participant one was a male aged 65.6 years, diagnosed 54 months prior to the study. Participant two was a female aged 49.6 years, diagnosed 24 months prior to the study. Participant symptoms presented at 66 and 33 months from the time of the study, respectively.

The objectives of the pilot study was to (i) finalize the measuring instruments; (ii) determine the equipment to be used in the study; (iii) determine the need for adaptation of test equipment; and (iv) determine the total testing time per participant. The results of the pilot study were then used to refine the methodology and to reduce the threats to internal and external validity (Teijlingen et al., 2001).

Main Study

Once participants were identified they were provided with the informed consent forms, the HEQ and HHIA prior to their scheduled appointment. Biological calibration of the equipment took place prior to participant arrival on the day of testing to ensure consistency in test recordings were upheld for the duration of the data collection procedure. The informed consent forms and completed questionnaires (HEQ and HHIA) were returned by participants on the scheduled appointment day. All audiometric measures were performed in one session. Behavioural measures were conducted first followed by the electrophysiological measures. This sequence of testing ensured that procedures reliant on active responses were completed first ensuring participant fatigue did not influence the reliability of test findings. Verbal feedback was given at the completion of the assessment session. Written audiological reports summarizing the findings from the auditory evaluation were compiled and issued with a two-week turnaround time from date of assessment. All the data was encoded and captured at the end of each session after which it was checked for any capturing errors. Accuracy of data capturing was then validated by the inter-rater.

Reliability and Validity

Reliability

Reliability refers to the consistency and accuracy of a given measurement and determines whether or not a replica of the findings of the current study would be obtained if the same methodology were to be repeated (Schiavetti & Metz, 2002). Inter-rater reliability, the use of a detailed test protocol and the elimination of systematic errors all contributed the reliability of the study.

Inter-rater reliability was determined by involving two raters, the researcher and an independent rater, in the data analysis. Both raters were suitably qualified Speech Language Pathologists and Audiologists, each with six years clinical experience in the field of diagnostic audiology. The independent rater was only provided with minimal information regarding the aims of the research study in an effort to limit the bias in data interpretation. The normative data for the formulated test protocol was issued to this rater to ensure the normative data used for result interpretation remained uniform across both raters. Twenty-five percent of the audiological results and HHIA scores were reviewed by the independent rater. The interrater agreement was 93.7%. Subjective assessment procedures further threatened the reliability of the current study. Non-interactional observer bias suggests misrepresentation in the documentation and/or interpretation of test results (Silverman, 2000). A detailed test protocol with equipment, procedures and instructions specified were followed during data collection to limit researcher subjectivity. Systematic errors, or evidence of measurement errors consistently reoccurring with each repeated measurement (Schiavetti & Metz, 2002), were eliminated by ensuring that all the audiological equipment used in the study were calibrated prior to the commencement of the study.

Validity

The internal validity of this study was ensured through equipment calibration that met the minimum standards defined by the South Africa Bureau of Standards as well as biologic calibration prior to the testing of each participant. Face validity of the case history questionnaire and the HEQ were established by a qualified audiologist with six years clinical experience who reviewed these measures. A pilot study was then conducted to further strengthen external validity.

Data Analysis and Statistical Procedures

Data was documented on all the relevant measuring instruments and encoded according to data definitions. Using Statistica software (StatSoft, 2005) the mean, standard deviation and Pearson's product-moment correlation were calculated. A 0.05 significance level was used for all statistical tests, unless specified otherwise.

RESULTS

Audiological Profile

The audiological profile will include a description of participant-reported auditory symptoms, as well as findings from audiological test battery (otoscopic examination, acoustic immitance measures, pure tone audiometry, speech audiometry, DPOAEs and neurodiagnostic ABR).

Audiological Symptoms

A range of audiological symptoms were described by participants and included tinnitus, difficulty listening in noise and hyperacusis. Five participants reported tinnitus and difficulty listening in noisy environments. Four participants reported hyperacusis and a further three participants complained of recruitment. Two participants reported dizziness and a history of ear discharge, while one indicated isolated experiences of hearing fluctuation, vertigo and a history of ear pain. While the majority of the auditory symptoms reported by participants were typical and representative of the nature of their hearing impairment, it is interesting to note that participants who reported hyperacusis were able to isolate the onset of hyperacusis to have followed the diagnosis of ALS. Exact time frames of the onset of hyperacusis were not however reliably acquired. These participants expressed particular concern with common sounds such as that of passing vehicles and barking of the neighbourhood dog to be a distressing and uncomfortable listening experience. Whilst this is not a reflection of the majority of participants, it is important that this is highlighted based on its unanticipated presentation. While evidence of hyperacusis remains anecdotal, this data invites itself to further exploration and research.

Otoscopic Findings

Otoscopic evaluation revealed clear ear canals, intact tympanic membranes and a visible cone of light in all but one ear. One participant presented with soft wax partially occluding the right ear canal.

Acoustic Immitance

Tympanometry

All participants presented with a Type A tympanogram bilaterally suggestive of pressure (+50daPa to – 150daPa), static compliance (0. 28 – 1. 8 cm^3) and ear canal volume (0. 2 – 2. 0 cm^3) within the normal range (Hall & Mueller, 1997). Table 2 provides an outline of results obtained through tympanometric measures along with the average, range and SD for pressure, compliance and ear canal volume for both the left and the right ears.

Table 2. Summary of Tympanometry Data with Average, Range and SD

Participants	Pressure (in daPa)		Compliance (in cm^3)		Volume (in cm^3)	
	Left ear	Right ear	Left ear	Right ear	Left ear	Right ear
P1	-30	-18	0. 28	0. 82	1. 2	1. 16
P2	-22	-40	0. 44	0. 31	0. 9	0. 92
P3	-32	-32	0. 89	0. 82	0. 98	0. 98
P4	-29	-64	0. 52	0. 45	0. 88	0. 75
P5	-27	-27	0. 9	0. 71	1. 14	1. 16
P6	-35	-40	0,86	0. 28	0. 88	1. 2
P7	-24	-42	0. 51	0. 37	1. 23	1. 04
P8	-32	-25	0. 48	0. 88	1. 04	1. 2
Average	-28. 9	-36. 0	0. 61	0. 58	1. 03	1. 05
Range	-28. 9–22	-64 -18	0.28–0.90	0.28– 0.88	0.88-1.23	0.75–1.20
SD	4. 4	14. 1	0. 24	0. 25	0. 14	0. 16

Acoustic Reflexes

Ipsilateral Reflexes

Ipsilateral acoustic reflex results are outlined in Table 3. All 16 ears presented with acoustic reflexes within the 70-90dBSPL range across the 500Hz-2000Hz range of ipsilateral reflexes. Absent reflexes were identified at 4000Hz ipsilaterally in six ears specifically for P1, P6 and P7 bilaterally.

Table 3. Summary of Ipsilateral Reflex Data with Average, Range and SD (N=16 ears)

	Ipsilateral reflexes (in dB)							
	Right ear				Left ear			
	500Hz	**1000Hz**	**2000Hz**	**4000Hz**	**500Hz**	**1000Hz**	**2000Hz**	**4000Hz**
P1	85	90	90	Absent	95	100	85	Absent
P2	95	90	95	100	90	95	90	100
P3	105	105	105	110	90	90	85	85
P4	105	95	105	105	95	95	100	100
P5	95	100	100	110	95	90	90	110
P6	105	100	100	Absent	100	105	100	Absent
P7	100	105	105	Absent	100	100	105	Absent
P8	100	95	100	105	100	105	100	105
Ave	98. 7	97. 5	100. 0	106	95. 6	97. 5	94. 4	100
Range	85–105	90–105	90–105	100-110	90–100	90–105	85–105	85–110
SD	6. 9	6. 0	5. 3	4. 2	4. 2	6. 0	7. 8	9. 4

Contralateral Reflexes

All ears (N = 16) presented with acoustic reflexes within the 70-90dBSPL range across the 500Hz-2000Hz range of contralateral reflexes. Table 4 provides contralateral reflex levels for eight participants and sixteen ears. Absent reflexes were recorded at 2000Hz in two ears specifically the right ear of P6 and the left ear of P7. Bilateral absent reflexes were noted at 4000Hz in five participants (P1, P5, P6, P7 and P8).

Table 4. Summary of Contralateral Reflex Data with Average, Range and SD (N=16 ears)

	Contralateral reflexes (in dB)							
	Right ear				Left ear			
	500Hz	**1000Hz**	**2000Hz**	**4000Hz**	**500Hz**	**1000Hz**	**2000Hz**	**4000Hz**
P1	90	95	90	Absent	105	110	110	Absent
P2	95	90	90	95	90	95	95	105
P3	105	105	95	95	100	100	105	105
P4	105	105	105	100	95	100	100	100
P5	95	100	110	Absent	105	110	110	Absent
P6	105	100	Absent	Absent	105	105	110	Absent
P7	105	110	105	Absent	105	110	Absent	Absent
P8	95	95	110	Absent	100	105	110	Absent
Average	99	100	100. 7	96. 6	100. 6	104. 3	105. 7	103. 3
Range	90 – 105	90 – 110	90 – 110	95 - 105	100-105	105-110	105–110	100–105
SD	6. 2	6. 5	8. 9	2. 9	5. 6	5. 6	6. 0	2. 9

Pure Tone Audiometry

The pure tone audiometry results for 16 ears will be presented in this section. The presented information will initially focus on findings of ear symmetry and laterality. A review of pure tone audiometry results for both air and bone conduction measures will follow. These findings will be reviewed in relation to the configuration, severity and type of hearing loss identified.

Laterality and Symmetry

Bilateral presentation of hearing was recorded for all participants. Symmetrical hearing patterns were identified for six participants. Two participants (P3 and P6) presented with an asymmetrical hearing pattern, marked by a >10dB difference between ear PTAs.

Air and Bone Conduction

The results revealed high frequency hearing loss in six participants. The severity of the loss varied amongst participants. A total of 12 ears tested presented with hearing impairment isolated to the high frequencies. Two participants (P2 and P3) presented with normal hearing bilaterally, although it must be noted that P3 presented with a large air-bone gap in the right ear despite normal hearing thresholds. Table 5 outlines the average, range and *SD* per frequency tested. PTAs are provided in Table 6. PTA values fall within the range of normal hearing (0 – 25dB) (Hall & Mueller, 1997). PTA is typically calculated based on the 500Hz, 1000Hz and 2000Hz frequency threshold average and therefore does not take into account high frequency hearing (Harrell, 2002). All individuals with exception to P2 and P3, who presented with normal hearing bilaterally, presented with a high frequency hearing impairment not detected by PTA calculations.

Table 5. Air Conduction Average, Range and SD

		Air conduction thresholds (in dB)							
		250Hz	**500Hz**	**1000Hz**	**2000Hz**	**3000Hz**	**4000Hz**	**6000Hz**	**8000Hz**
Ave	R ear	11.9	13.75	13.75	14.3	25.0	24.4	40.0	46.35
	L ear	10.6	11.25	10. 6	18. 1	36.7	30.0	46.0	44.4
Range	R ear	0 – 25	5-25	5 – 25	5 – 30	5 – 45	5 – 50	25 – 60	10 – 70
	L ear	0 – 25	5 – 20	5 – 25	5 – 30	30 – 45	0 – 55	25 – 70	-5 – 70
SD	R ear	10.3	6.9	8.3	10.8	20.0	15.2	16.4	19.4
	L ear	9.0	6.	7.8	11.0	7.6	18.3	16.4	26.7

Note*:* R represents the right ear and L represents the left ear.

Type of Hearing Loss

A total of six participants presented with bilateral sensorineural hearing impairment. Two participants (P2 and P3) presented with hearing within the normal threshold range bilaterally. P3 presented with a large air-bone gap in the right ear, however thresholds for both air and bone remained within the range of normal hearing. P3 was the only participant to present with a diagnosis of bulbar onset ALS; however the presence of the air-bone gap in the right ear may also be attributed to the presence of a partial wax occlusion in the right ear canal. Table 7 provides the range, average and SD.

Table 6. Pure Tone Average (PTA)

Participants	PTA (in dB)	
	Right	**Left**
P1	23. 3	16. 6
P2	8. 3	6. 6
P3	23. 3	6. 6
P4	6. 6	8. 3
P5	25	25
P6	11. 6	25
P7	5	8. 3
P8	8. 3	10
Average	15	20
Range	5 -31. 6	6. 6 – 26. 6
SD	14.1	8. 7

Table 7. Bone Conduction Average, Range and SD

		Bone conduction thresholds (in dB)				
		250Hz	**500Hz**	**1000Hz**	**2000Hz**	**4000Hz**
Average	R ear	5. 6	7. 5	5. 0	11.9	16. 9
	L ear	3. 1	8. 1	4. 4	15. 0	20. 6
Range	R ear	-5 – 20	-10 – 25	-5 – 25	0 – 30	-5 – 35
	L ear	-10 – 20	-5 – 20	0 – 15	5 – 30	-5 – 45
SD	R ear	8.2	11.3	11.6	10.7	13.9
	L ear	10.7	9.2	5.0	9.3	16.6

Note: R represents the right ear and L represents the left ear.

Configuration of Hearing Loss

The Majority of Participants (N = 12 Ears) Presented with a Sloping Configuration of Hearing Loss.

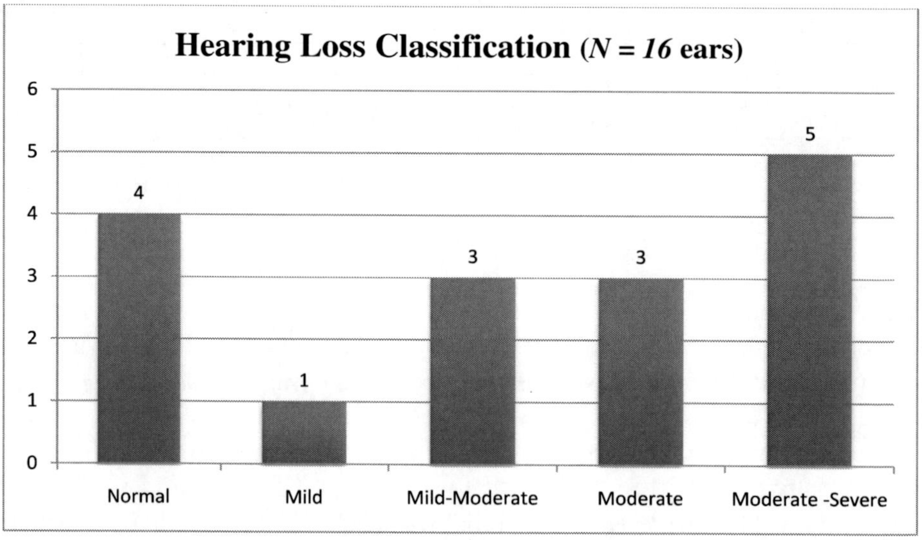

Figure 1. Hearing Loss Classification (N =16).

Degree of Hearing Loss

Figure 1 outlines the severity of the hearing loss of all participants with ALS (N = 16 ears). All the ears presented with normal hearing (0 -25dBHL) in the low-mid frequency range, consequently presenting with normal PTAs. The isolation of hearing loss to the 4000-8000Hz range limited the value of PTA scores which tend to be isolated to the low-mid frequency range. Applying a two-frequency calculation of PTA furthermore failed to represent the hearing loss accurately. The severity classification below is thus based on high frequency hearing thresholds, the region where 12 of the 16 ears presented with hearing impairment. The four remaining ears presented with normal hearing thresholds across the frequency range.

A total of four ears tested presented with normal hearing thresholds. One ear presented with a mild high frequency loss, followed by three who presented with a mild-moderate hearing impairment in the high frequencies. Three ears presented with a moderate high frequency hearing loss, while the remaining five ears, presented with a moderate – severe hearing loss in the high frequencies.

Table 8. Speech Audiometry Average, Range and SD

		Speech Audiometry (in dB)						
		SRT	**MCL**	**TD**	**DR**	**Sd (%)/ SRT+5dB**	**Sd (%) / SRT+25dB**	**Sd (%)/ TD - 10dB**
Ave	R ear	21.3	58.8	85.6	64.4	59.6	91.3	96.3
	L ear	21.9	56.9	86.3	64.4	44.6	90.6	94.9
Range	R ear	5 – 35	40 – 70	70 – 100	45 - 80	38-82	80 – 100	90 - 100
	L ear	10 – 60	40 – 70	70 – 105	20 - 90	0 - 79	77 – 100	85 - 100
SD	R ear	10.9	8.8	9.4	12.4	17.3	7.8	4.6
	L ear	16.0	10.7	11.3	19.4	28.5	8.9	5.8

Note: R represents the right ear and L represents the left ear.
Sd: Speech discrimination.

Speech Audiometry

These results include findings from speech reception thresholds (SRT), most comfortable levels (MCL), threshold of discomfort (TD), dynamic range (DR) and speech discrimination (Sd) testing (See Table 8).

Speech Reception Threshold

Speech reception in normal hearing individuals typically presents at 25dB sensation level (SL) (Brandy, 2001). Thirteen ears presented with SRT scores representative of the normal range (Table 24). In total, three ears presented with SRT scores outside the normative range. P5 experienced difficulty with SRT testing particularly for the left ear, where a SRT of 60 dBHL was recorded. This is a marked discrepancy when reviewed against a PTA of 25 dB in the corresponding ear. P7 presented with a SRT of 35 dBHL in the right ear further showing discrepancy between the PTA of 5 dB obtained for the same ear.

Most Comfortable Level

The MCL fell within the normative data range of 40 – 60 dBHL for all participants.

Threshold of Discomfort

TD levels typically present within the 80 – 100 dBHL for individuals with normal hearing (Thibodeau, 2007). TD averages fell within the normative data range, with the right ear average of 85.6 dBHL and the left ear average of 83.6 dBHL (Table 8). P6 and P7 were however noted to present with TDs at 70 dBHL in the right and left ears respectively, which falls below the normative range of discomfort levels. This suggests sensitivity to increased loudness intensity (Thibodeau, 2007). Discomfort levels below 85 dBHL are reported to be indicative of varying severity levels of hyperacusis (Vernon, 2002). These are evident for P2 left, P3 right, P5 right and P6 bilaterally all of whom reported complaints of hyperacusis. P7 also presented with TD below 85 dBHL in the left ear, however this is not paired with individual reports of hyperacusis.

Dynamic Range

These results are typically noted to present above 60dBHL in instances of normal hearing (Thibodeau, 2007). An average DR of 63.1 dBHL and 63.8 dBHL was recorded in the right and left ears respectively for all the participants (Table 8). These fall within the lower range of acceptable dynamic scores. Five ears presented with DR scores below the 60 dBHL minimum. This was observed in the right ear for P6 and bilaterally for P5 and P7. These scores are suggestive of recruitment and support the presence of cochlear pathology (Thibodeau, 2007).

Speech Discrimination

In normal hearing subjects, speech discrimination scores are anticipated to reach between 88 – 100% at the level of SRT +25dB. Scores below this are associated with a conductive or sensorineural (cochlear or retrocochlear) pathology. Rollover is not typically expected in normal hearing cases and is more highly associated with sensorineural hearing impairments. A rollover percentage of less than 20% supports the presence of cochlear site of lesion, while a rollover percentage greater than 20% provides evidence of retrocochlear pathology (Brandy, 2001). Scores typically revealed improved speech discrimination abilities at increasing intensity levels. Average scores for right and left ears support the speech discrimination abilities expected of individuals with normal hearing (Table 8). However, examination of individual ears revealed that three ears achieved percentage scores below the 88% minimum at SRT + 25dB supporting some extent of hearing impairment. This was identified for the left ear of P1 and the right ears for P5 and P6. Participant averages at TD – 10dB were 96.3 dBHL and 94.9 dBHL in the right and left ears respectively. These averages, when compared with SRT + 25dB averages do not suggest the presence of rollover. These findings support the presence of cochlear pathology.

A small difference of 4.9% and 4.3% can be observed between SRT+25 dB and TD-10 dB averages for the right and left ears respectively. It is important to note that many participants presented with hearing impairment isolated only to the high frequency region of 6000-8000Hz, while a majority of speech sounds fall within the 2000-4000Hz range. Speech discrimination scores suggested discrimination abilities within the normal range at

SRT+25dB even though hearing impairments were identified for all, but two participants in the sample. The presence of high frequency hearing impairment limited to the 6000-8000Hz range may account for these discrepancies.

Distortion Product OAEs

The average results obtained for DPOAE measures are outlined in Table 9. Based on the averages provided, it is evident that DPOAE amplitudes were present across the low-mid frequency ranges of 750Hz-1500Hz, while an increase in abnormal outer hair cell function was documented for high frequency ranges 2000-8000Hz. These averages represent a gradual decline in distortion product amplitude outside the >10 dB norm applied to this study in relation to increasing pure tone frequency. Signal-to-noise ratio (SNR) is considered as a means of differentiating impaired versus normal DPOAEs, although more specifically may be used as a means of determining the reliability of the DPOAE levels measured (Gorga, Neely, Dorn & Hoover, 2003). A SNR of >6 dB was achieved consistently throughout the frequency range with exception to those high frequency ranges of 6000Hz – 8000Hz. Absent DPOAEs were recorded in the left ear at 8000Hz for P6 and P7 at 6000-8000Hz in the left ear. The remaining participants all obtained DPOAEs, although not all of these were normal emissions. P2 and P3 presented with normal hearing thresholds and acquired DPOAE recordings that corresponded with all emissions were recorded across the frequency range with a SNR above 6dB. The remaining participants achieved emissions across the frequencies ranging from 750Hz-4000Hz, while SNR showed deterioration in the 6000Hz-8000Hz range. Abnormal DPOAEs in this frequency region is suggestive of impaired functioning of the outer hair cells of the cochlea, isolating the cochlea as the potential site of lesion.

Table 9. DPOAE Frequency Specific Average, Range and SD

			DPOAE Averages (in dB)							
		Ear	750Hz	1000Hz	1500Hz	2000Hz	3000Hz	4000Hz	6000Hz	8000Hz
Amplitude	Ave	R	12. 1	11. 3	11. 7	9. 8	9. 6	9. 5	7. 0	5. 8
		L	11. 8	11. 1	10. 3	8. 2	9. 5	7. 9	5. 8	0
	Range	R	10. 0–15. 3	4. 4–16. 8	9. 2– 8. 0	5. 2– 3. 3	6. 4– 1. 2	3. 9 – 4. 3	4. 3 – 3. 3	3. 5 – 3. 4
		L	10. 1 –6. 0	8. 3 –15. 0	7. 7 –11. 6	0. 0 –11. 4	4. 6 –14. 2	-7. 8 –14. 5	-0. 9 -12. 4	-12. 2–13. 9
	SD	R	2. 0	3. 5	2. 7	2. 8	1. 8	3. 6	3. 2	3. 3
		L	1. 9	2. 0	1. 3	3. 7	4. 0	4. 6	6. 6	9. 8
SNR	Ave	R	8. 75	8. 09	8. 9	7. 2	7. 8	8. 3	5. 6	4. 4
		L	7. 3	8. 1	7. 9	9. 1	9. 6	8. 1	6. 8	3. 1
	Range	R	6. 5 –10. 8	6 – 15. 7	6. 3 - 18	6. 1 – 8. 9	6 – 12. 6	4. 4 –19. 6	-5. 5 –13. 3	-2 – 7. 6
		L	6. 3 –10. 2	6. 1 –13. 9	6. 1 –10. 2	6. 8 –15. 7	3. 5 –15. 8	1. 5 –16. 5	-1. 8 –16. 5	-5. 8 – 7. 2
	SD	R	2. 7	3. 3	3. 8	1. 0	2. 1	4. 7	5. 2	2. 9
		L	1. 2	2. 6	1. 6	3. 0	4. 6	4. 7	6. 2	5. 3

Note: Ave (average); *SD* (standard deviation); R (right); L (left); SNR (signal to noise ratio).

A high correlation between DPOAE and audiometric thresholds is typically noted in the mid-high frequency range (Gorga et al., 2003). This is supported in these findings whereby DPOAE SNRs correspond with the increasing loss of hearing in the high frequency range. Outer hair cell function is isolated to approximately 50 – 60 dB hearing loss resulting in less reliable DPOAE recordings as hearing loss approaches these threshold levels (Bartnik et al., 2009). The increase in hearing loss noted in the high frequencies resulted in a SNR falling below the 6dB range suggesting outer hair cell damage in the range of 50-60 dB and beyond.

Pearson's product moment correlation was applied to the data to best determine correlations. DPOAE testing revealed moderately positive correlations between all consecutive frequencies tested, namely 1000Hz and 1500Hz, 2000Hz and 3000Hz, 4000Hz and 6000Hz and 6000Hz and 8000Hz. These correlation coefficients ranged from 0.51 – 0.69, while strong positive correlations were revealed for 6000Hz and 8000Hz (r = 0.93). Moderately negative correlations were identified between pure tone audiometry and DPOAE measures at 1000Hz, 2000Hz and 4000Hz. These correlation coefficients ranged between R = -0.59 to -0.73, while strong negative correlations at 6000Hz and 8000Hz ranged between R = -0.89 to -0.91. Ongoing consideration for the low number of data points applied to these analyses prevents generalization of these findings.

Neurodiagnostic ABR

The summary of neurodiagnostic ABR results are outlined in Table 10. When applying a SD of 0.2 msec to inter peak latencies (IPL) normative data (95% confidence interval) suggests that only I-III and III-V IPLs exceeding 2. 2 msec and IPLs I-V exceeding 4. 2 msec are considered abnormal (Don & Kwong, 2002). As is evident in Table 10, IPL averages were within the normal range for all participant ears in the current study (N = 16) and did not exceed the time frame outlined in the protocol applied to this study. Absolute wave latencies (AWL) for wave I, III and V were present at 1.6 msec, 3.6 msec and 5.6 msec (SD of 0.2msec; 95% confidence interval) in individuals without retrocochlear pathology (Don & Kwong, 2002). The averages calculated for participants in the current study reflect these norms accordingly with AWL for waves I, III and V not exceeding these parameters. Inspection of each case in isolation brings to light a number of factors that are not revealed when reviewing combined test averages.

IPL for wave I-V fall within the normal range (4. 0 msec with 0.2 msec SD). P2 and P5 present with slightly shorter wave I–V IPLs. Five participants (P1, P4, P5 bilaterally, P3 right, P6 left) and eight ears (50%) presented with longer wave I-III IPLs, while the remaining participants presented with I-III IPLs within the normative range. The five participants presenting with slightly delayed IPLs also presented with the more severe high frequency hearing impairment. All participants presented with wave III-V IPLs that were shorter than the outlined normative range (1.8 – 2.2 msec).

The AWL for waves I, III and V for all the participants were within normal limits, although slightly shorter latencies were consistently noted particularly for wave I and V AWL recordings. The shorter latencies identified throughout AWL measurements may be associated with the selection of a rarefaction polarity, which typically present with shorter latencies of 0.1 – 0.2 msec from the normal range (Don & Kwong, 2002).

An interaural wave latency differences (IAWLD) for wave V of >0.4 msec is associated with retrocochlear pathology (Hall & Mueller, 1997). It is evident from Table 10 that the IAWLD for all participants were within normal limits (average = 0.11 msec). It can thus be concluded that based on the results of the neurodiagnostic ABR test, that none of the participants presented with auditory neuropathy or pathology at the site of the brainstem.

These findings correlate with pure tone audiometry and speech discrimination results, which through the absence of >20% rollover for the total sample further eliminated any audiometric indicators of a retrocochlear site of lesion. These findings, when interpreted with DPOAE results, suggest that where SNHL is indicated, a cochlear site of lesion is most probable for the majority of participants in the current study.

Table 10. Summary of raw neurodiagnostic ABR data with Average, Range and SD

	Ear	Interpeak latency (IPL) (in msec)			Absolute Wave Latency (AWL) (in msec)			IAWLD of Wave V (in msec)
		Waves I-III	Waves III-V	Waves I-V	Wave I	Wave III	Wave V	
P1	L	2.3	1.6	3.87	1.33	3.6	5.2	0.13
	R	2.3	1.7	4.0	1.33	3.6	5.33	
P2	L	2.0	1.67	3.67	1.2	3.2	4.87	0.0
	R	1.9	1.65	3.54	1.33	3.22	4.87	
P3	L	2.1	1.67	3.87	1.3	3.4	5.1	0.17
	R	2.3	1.67	3.93	1.33	3.6	5.27	
P4	L	2.3	1.78	4.11	1.27	3.6	5.38	0.18
	R	2.3	1.6	3.87	1.33	3.6	5.2	
P5	L	2.4	1.27	3.67	1.2	3.6	4.87	
	R	2.3	1.37	3.64	1.33	3.6	4.97	0.10
P6	L	2.3	1.73	4.0	1.33	3.6	5.33	0.23
	R	2.0	1.77	3.8	1.3	3.33	5.1	
P7	L	2.0	1.77	3.77	1.33	3.33	5.1	0.1
	R	1.7	1.78	3.9	1.3	3.42	5.2	
P8	L	2.1	1.7	3.73	1.29	3.4	5.1	0.00
	R	2.2	1.56	3.73	1.37	3.54	5.1	
Ave	L	2.17	1.64	3.83	1.28	3.46	5.12	0.11
	R	2.10	1.64	3.80	1.31	3.28	5.13	
Range	L	2 – 2.4	1.27– .78	3.67– .0	1.2 – 1.33	3.2 – 3.6	4.87 – 5.38	0 – 0.23
	R	1. 72 - 2.27	1. 37– 1.78	3.54– 4.0	1.27 – 1.33	3.22 – 3.6	4.87 – 5.33	
SD	L	0.15	0.16	0.16	0.05	0.16	0.19	0.08
	R	0.21	0.13	0.16	0.02	0.15	0.15	

Perceptions of Auditory Impairment

The second aim of the study was to explore the perceptions of individuals with ALS and their caregivers of the implications of auditory impairment and value of auditory diagnosis.

Perceived Psychosocial Implications of Hearing Loss on Daily Functioning

This section will present the findings from the HHIA inventory related to socially and emotionally perceived implications of hearing loss. It will in addition explore the relation between the HHIA and audiometric test measures obtained for participants in this study. This section will then conclude with a review of participant responses to the HEQ and participant and caregiver perceptions related to the value of auditory testing and diagnosis alongside the ALS.

HHIA Review

The HHIA reviews individual hearing experience on both a social and an emotional scale to ascertain the psychosocial level of functioning of the hearing impaired individual (Newman et al., 1990). Participant scores are added resulting in a handicap classification of 'none', suggesting no handicap related to hearing impairment or 'mild', suggesting limited effects of hearing impairment on social and emotional wellbeing. A 'moderate' score suggests limited or average success in functional activities related to hearing ability, whilst a 'severe' score is indicative of critically harmful effects on individual social and emotional wellbeing as a result of hearing impairment (Newman et al., 1990). Participant responses to the HHIA are outlined in Table 11, followed by a statistical review of the correlation between participant auditory test findings and the associated emotional and/or social implications thereof.

The results indicate that four of the participants reported no auditory handicap. Two participants reported a mild hearing handicap, while two participants reported a moderate hearing handicap impacting social and/or emotional functionality. Only two participants acknowledged hearing difficulties in the initial case history interview, with the remaining six reporting no auditory impairment.

The HHIA scale revealed wide variation in scores across participants, ranging from no reported handicap to moderate reported handicap. Four participants (P1, P3, P6 and P8) reported greater handicap at a level of social functioning over emotional wellbeing. One participant (P7) reported greater handicap at a level of emotional functioning. Three participants reported no differences between emotional and social functioning, of whom two (P2 and P4) presented with no handicap and one participant (P5) presented with a moderate handicap on the HHIA.

Correlation analysis for social versus emotional participant responses was performed using Pearson's product moment correlation coefficient. A 0.05 significance level was used for this statistical measure. The social versus the emotional responses showed good correlation ($r = 0.86$; $p = 0.006$) suggesting participants with higher social handicap typically were noted to have higher emotional handicap scores as well. Across the entire sample, ALS participants responded '*yes*' to 12.5% (12 responses) of the twelve social questions, while a response of '*sometimes*' was associated with 15.6% (15 responses) of these questions. The remaining 71.9% of participant responses indicated that participants did not associate with the remaining social handicaps outlined in the HHIA. A total of 7.69% (8 responses) out of thirteen questions linked to the emotional effects of hearing impairment received '*yes*' responses from participants, while a response of '*sometimes*' was associated with an additional 11.5% (12 responses) of the thirteen questions. The remaining 80.81% of participant responses indicated that participants did not experience the remaining emotional handicaps outlined by the HHIA.

Despite the good correlation between social and emotional scores, the percentage of positive scores from the HHIA suggests that the social implications of hearing impairment appear to be more readily acknowledged and reported than those at an emotional level. Participants reporting occasional difficulties in certain domains may represent the total of the sample experiencing initial markers suggestive of hearing impairment and/or denial related to the vast range and extent of deterioration in bodily function brought about by ALS.

Difficulties experienced in different contexts were also probed. Four participants agreed that they experience social difficulty in a restaurant setting. Two participants reported difficulties in social activities including telephone use, listening success in movies, and television or radio use. One participant indicated that difficulty with telephone use and listening in movies was 'sometimes' problematic. Three participants indicated television and radio use to be an occasional area of difficulty, alongside difficulties in loud noise situations e.g. party/ social groups. The latter was met with firm agreement by two participants.

Table 11. HHIA participant response (N = 8)

Q	Nature	Content of Question	P1	P2	P3	P4	P5	P6	P7	P8
1	Social	Less phone use	Y	N	N	N	N	Y	S	N
2	Emotional	Embarrassment	N	N	N	N	N	N	N	N
3	Social	Group Avoidance	N	N	N	N	S	Y	N	N
4	Emotional	Irritability	S	N	N	N	S	S	Y	N
5	Emotional	Family Frustration	S	N	N	N	N	N	Y	N
6	Social	Difficulty at Party/ Social Function	Y	S	N	N	S	N	S	N
7	Social	Understanding clients/coworker	S	N	N	N	S	N	N	N
8	Emotional	Handicap	N	N	N	N	N	N	N	N
9	Social	Difficulty visiting doctors, family	S	N	N	N	N	N	N	N
10	Emotional	Co-Worker Frustration	N	N	N	N	N	N	N	N
11	Social	Difficulty in Movie/Theater Setting	N	N	N	N	Y	Y	S	N
12	Emotional	Nervousness	N	N	N	N	N	N	N	N
13	Social	Less frequent visiting	N	N	N	N	S	Y	N	N
14	Emotional	Family Arguments	S	N	N	N	Y	N	S	N
15	Social	Difficulty TV/radio	S	N	N	N	Y	S	Y	S
16	Social	Less frequent shopping	N	N	N	N	N	N	N	N
17	Emotional	Difficulty hearing – upsetting	S	N	N	N	Y	Y	S	N
18	Emotional	Isolation/ Desire to be left alone	N	N	N	N	N	N	N	N
19	Social	Less frequent communication with family	N	N	N	N	N	S	N	N
20	Emotional	Hampers social life	S	N	N	N	Y	Y	S	N
21	Social	Difficulty in restaurants	Y	N	N	N	Y	S	Y	Y
22	Emotional	Cause depression	N	N	N	N	N	N	N	N
23	Social	Less frequent TV/radio use	N	N	N	N	N	N	N	N

Table 11. (Continued)

Q	Nature	Content of Question	P1	P2	P3	P4	P5	P6	P7	P8
24	Emotional	Discomfort communicating with friends	N	N	N	N	S	N	N	N
25	Emotional	Isolation when in social groups	S	N	Y	N	Y	N	S	N
		SOCIAL TOTAL	18	0	4	0	20	22	14	6
		EMOTIONAL TOTAL	12	0	0	0	20	10	16	0
		GRAND TOTAL	30	0	4	0	40	32	30	6
		HANDICAP RATING	MILD	NONE	NONE	NONE	MOD	MOD	MILD	NONE

Note: Y represents 'Yes' responses, N represents 'No' responses and S represents 'Sometimes' responses.

Table 12. Statistical Correlation between HHIA and Pure Tone Average

Category	*r*	*Correlations*
HHIA Social	0. 71	0.050*
HHIA Emotional	0. 63	0.095
HHIA Total	0. 70	0.056*

* Significant at the 90% confidence level.

At an emotional level the most common participant concerns were related to items 17, 20 and 25 where hearing difficulties were identified to be 'upsetting', a hindrance to social activity and result in isolation from groups of people respectively. In these instances, two participants positively identified with these difficulties, with a further two participants reporting occasional difficulties in each of the above listed instances.

HHIA and Auditory Testing

A comparative review of the recorded HHIA responses and the auditory findings (PTA and speech audiometry) was executed as a means of determining the psychosocial impact of hearing impairment in the functioning of the participants in this study. Pearson's product moment correlation coefficient was used as the statistical measure for the review of HHIA findings and pure tone averages, with a confidence interval of 0.05.

HHIA and Pure Tone Average

Statistical review of the correlation between PTA averages against HHIA social scores are indicative of a relatively strong, positive correlation ($r = 0.71; p = 0.050$) (Table 12). This suggests that for those participants presenting with higher pure tone averages, (i.e. poorer auditory abilities), the level of reported handicap at a social level of functioning increased. A poorer correlation was observed between pure tone averages and HHIA emotional handicap ratings ($r = 0.63; p = 0.095$). It is postulated that individuals with ALS in this study do not readily acknowledge or report the emotional implications of hearing loss (e.g. feelings of embarrassment, self-isolation, nervousness and/or perception of auditory handicap), despite audiometric evidence of hearing impairment. Review of the total HHIA scores revealed a positive correlation (*r = 0.69; p = 0.056),* indicating that the higher the total pure tone average, the higher the total HHIA level of handicap are.

The PTA revealed moderately positive correlations with social and total HHIA scores and a poor correlation for emotional handicap ratings. Pure tone audiometry is therefore an adequate indicator of the level of auditory impact at a social level for individuals with ALS although the limited sample size precludes the identification of any strong, definitive trends.

HHIA and Speech Audiometry

The correlation between the average speech discrimination scores and the HHIA totals revealed significant negative correlation of r = -0.74 (p = 0.034). This suggests that an increase in speech discrimination abilities corresponded with lower HHIA scores. The correlation between speech discrimination and social HHIA rating revealed a significant negative correlation of r = -0.74 (p = 0.038), while emotional ratings from the HHIA supported a negative correlation of marginal significance (r = -0.70; p = 0054).

Hearing Experience Questionnaire (HEQ)

The HEQ were completed by both individuals with ALS and their caregivers. Individuals with ALS completed three sections, namely (i) contact with the discipline of speech pathology and/or audiology, (ii) rating functional skills in order of importance, and (iii) the importance of receiving an auditory diagnosis. Caregivers only completed the last two sections indicated above.

Contact with Speech Pathology and/or Audiology

Of all the participants, only two participants (P3 and P5) had attended consultations with a speech pathologist at the onset of ALS to facilitate augmentative and alternative communication. None of the participants in this study reported contact with an audiologist, or had been referred for an auditory evaluation or undergone previous auditory examination. None of the participants reported receiving information on hearing loss or the effects this may have on quality of life from a speech-language pathologist, audiologist or another professional in the medical management team. As participants in the current study voluntarily remained an average of 45 minutes following test time to address concerns related to auditory symptoms and discuss stressors related to auditory difficulties, this suggests a need for such support.

Functional Rating Scale

The categories of communication, arm movement, hearing, leg movement, vision, chewing and swallowing for nutrition were included in this section. Both individuals with ALS and their caregivers were required to rate various functional abilities according to their personal order of perceived importance when related to living with ALS. Figure 2 outlines participant and caregiver responses to this rating scale.

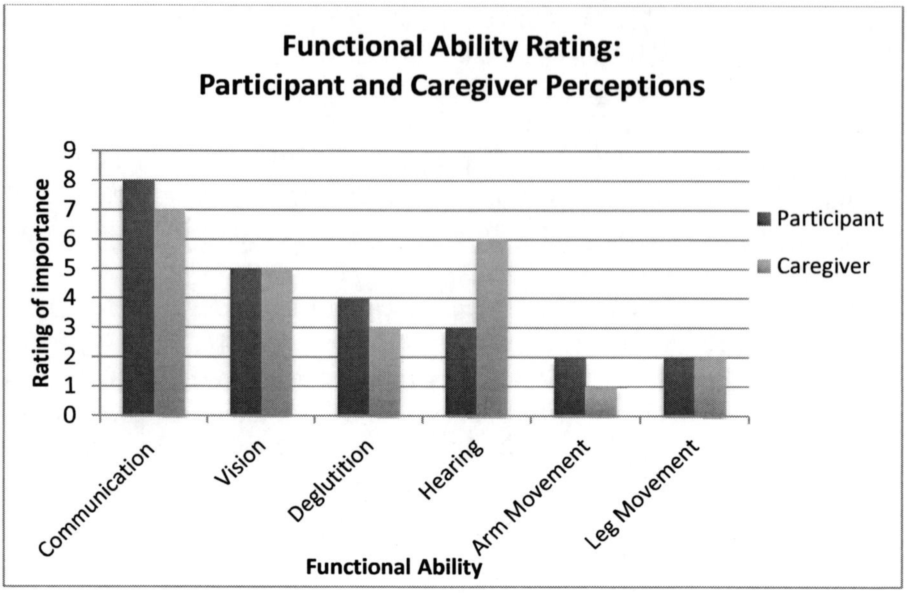

Figure 2. Functional Ability Rating: Participant and Caregiver Perceptions.

Results revealed variations in the perspective of individuals with ALS and their caregivers. Both individuals with ALS and their caregivers rated vision and leg movement similarly. Communication, deglutition, hearing and arm movement however presented with more differences in opinion. Amongst these differences, the rating of hearing ability presented with the greatest contrasting views between the two groups.

Communication rated very highly amongst both individuals with ALS and their caregivers. All eight individuals with ALS and seven caregivers identified communicative skills as a priority functional ability. The importance of communicative skills to participants was then followed by visual ability and deglutition. Arm and leg movement were not rated highly amongst participants, as participants indicated that adjustments to lifestyle can and in many instances have been made to accommodate the loss of these abilities. The general perception that communication and vision were central to maintaining contact with the 'outside world' was shared amongst participants, while deglutition was identified as the third critical functional domain being connected to a number of varying explanations and participant perspectives.

Participants in this study highlighted the connection between eating and maintenance of social wellbeing. Participants reported that swallowing difficulties were harmful to social opportunity and since most adult socialization occurs alongside dining activities a great deal of anxiety and distress is brought on. An inability eat/swallow in a socially respectful manner i.e. without coughing and choking on food, contributes to making one an undesirable social partner within these settings. Participants felt that swallowing difficulties in social settings were isolating and damaging to their self-esteem and dignity, more so than auditory impairment. When probed further regarding the option of non-oral feeding methods, these were also declined as a socially acceptable solution with suggestions that this gives rise to feelings of social exclusion. Participants were noted to associate deglutition very closely with social success.

Where participants rated visual ability to be the second most important requirement contributing to quality of daily living, caregivers interestingly rated hearing ability as a key ability that would have influence on the quality of life of their ALS spouse/partner. Hearing ability was viewed as important by six caregivers, in contrast to only three individuals with ALS. Visual ability rated third highest by both the individuals with ALS and their caregivers. Caregivers demonstrated a firm awareness of the benefits of preserved visual acuity related to the use of AAC devices and the use of these devices as a means of maintaining expressive communicative function. Arm and leg movement contributed to the lowest rating by caregivers, with leg movement rated as a marginally more important supporting the theme of adjustment and indicated that current technology allows for livable modifications to be successfully achieved overcoming difficulties with mobility.

Identifying Importance of Auditory Diagnosis

The last section of the HEQ, individuals with ALS and caregivers were questioned on the relevance an added diagnosis of hearing loss superimposed on the diagnosis of ALS would have. The majority of participants with ALS (n = 5) reported that the added diagnosis of hearing loss would be of no relevance to them. Hence, acquiring information about auditory function would not be pursued individually. Participant responses largely centered on the themes of burden and loss of sense of self. Participants indicated that the added diagnosis would have no positive impact on their quality of life. They expressed the viewpoint that gradually progressive deterioration of motor function was enough to deal with. A single participant acknowledged the need for ongoing research regarding the presentation of auditory symptoms in ALS. Two participants highlighted the importance of hearing in relation to the themes of autonomy, control and maintaining a sense of self in the face of ALS.

In contrast, the majority of caregivers (n = 5) viewed auditory diagnosis to be extremely important. They related this to the need for the individual with ALS to maintain a desirable quality of life through sustained autonomy and alleviation of individual and caregiver burden. Furthermore the need for maintaining individual involvement in social and community life as well as hobbies creating a sense of purpose (e.g. musical interests) were revealed. One caregiver indicated that information on auditory status of individuals with ALS would only be interesting for researchers. Two caregivers indicated that the added knowledge of hearing impairment would not have any significance, mostly as the additional cost of amplification will increase the financial burden as a consequence of ALS. They also highlighted that the emotional turmoil of adding further diagnosis to an already diagnostically untreatable degenerative disease serves no benefit to individual psychological and emotional wellbeing.

DISCUSSION

Hearing Loss and ALS

A review of the audiological findings provided an audiological of individual with ALS in the current study. Two participants (P2 and P3) presented with normal hearing thresholds bilaterally, while the majority of participants (n = 6) with varying extents of hearing loss isolated to the high frequencies. One of the participants with normal hearing (P3) presented with a large air-bone gap in the right ear despite borderline normal thresholds being recorded. Participant 3 was the only participant in the total sample to have a diagnosis of bulbar ALS. She also presented with a soft wax occlusion in the right ear alongside a history of ear discharge. Any of these factors in isolation and/or combination may be associated with the large air-bone gap.

In a study that investigated the differences in auditory thresholds ranging from 500Hz - 4000Hz before and after wax removal, it was found that hearing improved by an average of 5 dB across the frequency range analyzed (Sharp, Wilson, Ross, & Barr-Hamilton, 1990). This change in hearing ability, although small, may negate the need for amplification for an individual that is a borderline hearing aid candidate (Sharp et al., 1990). When a 5 dB improvement across the frequency range of P3's right hearing thresholds is applied the extent of the air-bone gap lessens, although remains relatively large with a 15-20dB gap between air and bone thresholds across the low – mid frequency range. This suggests that wax occlusion may not be the only factor contributing to this air-bone gap. Furthermore, P3 reported and demonstrated only mild consequences of infrequent recurrent infections during auditory testing thereby validating the borderline normal hearing thresholds recorded for the right ear. A history of ear infections has damaging effects on hearing levels later in life and typically has more harmful effects on quality of life amongst adult subjects in contrast to younger subjects (Tambs, 2004).

Interestingly, P3 was the only participant in the sample to present with a diagnosis of bulbar onset ALS, which may serve as an additional factor contributing to the increased air-bone gap. Bulbar onset ALS is typically characterized by motor neuron degeneration in the regions of the cerebral cortex, brainstem, spinal cord and the pyramidal tracts. These regions typically involve cranial nerves IX (glossopharyngeal), X (vagus) and XII (hypoglossal) (Snell, 2001). Further review into the innervations of the glossopharyngeal nerve reveals supply to the middle ear region. While the glossopharyngeal nerve carries largely sensory functions, a visceral motor component exists, exiting the inferior ganglion emerging as the tympanic nerve, serving the tympanic cavity of the middle ear (Snell, 2001). The involvement of this nerves' innervations to the middle ear region as well as its' relation to bulbar neuron degeneration highlights the need for further investigation into its' involvement in the onset of conductive hearing impairment in individuals diagnosed with bulbar onset ALS.

Conductive hearing loss in ALS may further be attributed to the paralysis of the tensor and levator veli palatini muscles. These muscles play a crucial role in controlling the mechanical properties of the Eustachian tube. Paralysis of these muscles, on account of motor neuron degeneration linked to bulbar symptoms, prevents the active dilation of the Eustachian tube resulting in increased lumen in these regions (Ghadiali et al., 2003). The outcome of such paralysis leads to the development of negative middle ear pressure, ultimately increasing individual risk for developing otitis media with discharge (Ghadiali et al., 2003). This hypothesis supports the presence of a large air-bone gap in P3's hearing thresholds and is supported when viewed in conjunction with reports of recurrent 'infrequent' ear infection presenting since ALS onset. Additionally, it is viable that thresholds remained within the normal limits, since the most recent occurance of discharge was reported to have occurred over 8 months prior to the test date. Therefore, since P3 did not display signs of active infection (discharge, pain, lack of tympanic membrane clarity) at the time of testing, test results reflected normal auditory abilities. Tympanometry measures were further indicative of normal functioning in the region of the middle ear, although this may be the result of active infection not being present at the time of testing, thereby having no negative effect on the middle ear pressure.

The majority of participants (n = 6) presented with varying extents of high frequency hearing loss. Review of all test results in combination support the presence of a high frequency hearing loss isolated to the region of the cochlea. Caution is however required in isolating the etiology of this hearing loss as a definitive factor related to ALS. The nature of the loss identified in this study corresponds to the pattern of presbycusis – a hearing loss arising as a result of the natural aging process (Dalton et al., 2003). This is of particular relevance since the onset of ALS (fourth to sixth decades of life), coincides with the onset of age related hearing impairment (48-87 years) (Dalton et al., 2003).

Presbycusis is characterized by loss or death of the hair cells of the inner ear and/or atrophy of the auditory nerve in the basal region of the cochlea, presenting as a SNHL (Weinstein, 2002). The onset is typically around middle age with a gradually progressive nature. Individuals with an age related hearing loss express a number of primary complaints, the foremost of which relates to difficulties discriminating speech in noise (Weinstein, 2002). This corresponds with the reports of P1, P4. P5, P7 and P8. Presbycusis may or may not co-occur with tinnitus, however this symptom was reported by five participants in the current study (P1, P4, P5, P7 and P8).

Tinnitus and hyperacusis frequently co-occur (Vesterager, 1997). Hyperacusis was reported to co-occur with tinnitus by four participants in the current study. The resultant increase in loudness perception reported amongst 50% of participants, further supports the cochlea as the primary site of lesion for hearing loss in ALS-participants in the current study. Presbycusis presents as a sloping loss where hearing thresholds are typically normal between 250Hz – 2000Hz, thus affecting the high frequencies first. These findings correspond to the pattern of hearing loss noted in P1, P4, P5, P6, P7 and P8 in the current study.

It is evident from the above description of presbycusis and its' related audiometric features, that the six participants in the current study who presented with bilateral sensorineural impairment presented with remarkable similarity in presentation to that of individuals with presbycusis. It is also relevant to note that while P2 did not present with hearing impairment, she was the youngest (49.6 years old) of all the participants. A 7.7 year age difference existed between P2 and the next participant when reviewed in increasing chronological order.

The onset of presbycutic audiometric signs may not yet be subjectively or objectively apparent at P2's age, as she is at the lower end of the age spectrum for presbycutic onset. It is furthermore documented that the hearing levels of males are typically poorer and difficulties present earlier than those of females, providing additional support for the absence of hearing loss in P2 at the time of the study, based on her gender and age (Weinstein, 2004). In conclusion, although hearing loss has been identified in the majority of the sample population, it is not possible to firmly conclude that the presence of hearing loss identified in this study exists primarily and definitively as a symptom of ALS. This is particularly due to the limited sample in this study.

The Perceptions of the Implications of Hearing Loss in Individuals with ALS

Hearing Handicap Inventory for Adults

The negative impact of hearing impairment on social and emotional wellbeing is well documented (Dalton et al., 2002). The severity of the hearing loss is positively associated with decreased function at a psychosocial level, which has greater implications in the ALS population due to the added physical deterioration further compounding activities of daily living and quality of life. The HHIA scale revealed wide variation in scores across participants in the current study, ranging from no reported handicap to moderate reported handicap. It is however important to bear in mind that all scores fall within the bottom 40% of the inventory scale. Caution must be exercised in the use of these findings as a reflection of the general ALS population due to the limited sample size and thus the limited power of generalizability.

It is interesting to note that while only two of participants initially reported some extent of hearing impairment, six presented hearing impairment as revealed through audiometric testing. Four participants also reported an auditory handicap on the HHIA. This demonstrates the discrepancy between initial reports of hearing impairment and audiometric findings; and between audiometric findings and perceived social and emotional handicap. These discrepancies are supported by the literature, which reveal that self- report measures typically underestimate the prevalence of hearing loss, resulting in the underreporting of hearing related difficulties (Dalton et al., 2003; Hallberg et al., 2008). It has been found that only 22% of individuals with a mild hearing loss, and 56% of individuals with a moderate-severe hearing loss, report a hearing handicap (Dalton et al., 2003). In contrast, 59% and 80% of individuals with mild and moderate-severe hearing losses respectively, isolated communication difficulties as a concern using the same self-report format. This suggests that individuals view communication difficulties to be of greater importance than auditory abilities, a notion further supported by individual opinions expressed in the HEQ for participants in the current study. Only two participants in the current study reported moderate difficulties related to hearing loss and socio-emotional factors. Nachtegaal et al. (2009) report that psychosocial health related to hearing impairment is reduced amongst older adults aged 65 years and older. The cut off age for this study was set at 66 years of age, thus it may be inferred that the low acknowledgement of hearing loss amongst the participants in this study is possibly a result of greater success at a psychosocial level than that of older adults.

Cross-sectional studies have revealed emotional disorders linked to anxiety and depression paired with ALS diagnosis (Goldstein & Leigh, 1999). This suggests that depression and low self-esteem have a direct relationship to the effects of ALS on everyday functioning and quality of life (Goldstein & Leigh, 1999). It may be additionally important to consider that the participants in the current study perceive emotional handicap to be more closely related to the diagnosis, progression and severity of neuro-degeneration rather than auditory impairment. The latter suggests that individuals associate socio-emotional handicap as a direct result of ALS, but fail to consider secondary or external impairments such as hearing ability. This validates the lower scores allocated to emotional hearing handicap ratings in the HHIA.

It is further postulated that self-deception regarding hearing loss is often adopted as a means of protecting individual identity and image (Hallberg, 1999). This is particularly true in instances where there is a discrepancy between one's reality and desired self-image.

Individuals with ALS deal with a steady and gradual loss of function placing emphasis on the need to constantly redefine self-image to match reality (McLeod & Clarke, 2007). In instances where individuals deal with an ongoing need for readjustment, denial and failure to acknowledge these difficulties occurs. Individuals may hence consciously or subconsciously underestimate the negative effects of hearing loss despite the external changes in communicative behaviors that arise as a direct consequence (Hallberg et al., 2008).

An additional explanation for HHIA responses revealing minimal socio-emotional concerns (with exception to P5 and P6) may relate to the extent of hearing impairment. Hearing loss across the entire sample was isolated to the high frequencies between 6000-8000Hz. It is possible that the frequency range affected by hearing loss is not yet broad enough to impose a more significant impact on the social and emotional functioning of the individual.

Hearing Experience Questionnaire (HEQ)

Contact with Speech Pathology and/or Audiology

At the time of the study, none of the participants had been referred for auditory testing, educated on auditory impairment or counseled regarding the effects of auditory impairment on quality of life. A study exploring the perspectives of services for ALS by individuals with ALS and their caregivers, revealed that while they praised the efforts made by members of the management teams, deficiencies in professional knowledge linked to ALS was highlighted (Brown, Lattimer & Tudball, 2006). In addition to this, the organization of secondary health services, counseling and emotional support to families and individuals with ALS emerged as limitations. Brown et al. (2006) conclude that emphasizing the quality of inter-professional and multi-agency co-operation is an important means of promoting and enhancing the quality of care given to individuals with ALS. Furthermore, knowledgeable care teams who consider primary and secondary consequences of ALS additionally contribute to enhancing the support, management and overall experience of living with ALS (Brown et al., 2006; Ward et al., 2003).

Findings of the current study cannot conclusively isolate hearing impairment to ALS despite the presentation of hearing impairment in the majority of participants. As the age of ALS onset, correspond with the onset of presbycusis, individuals with ALS may also present with hearing loss. It is therefore imperative that these individuals' hearing should be monitored throughout the course of the disease. It is postulated that this will serve to reduce the damaging effects of hearing loss on individual quality of life and ultimately the willingness to pursue life-prolonging measures (Ward et al., 2003).

Functional Rating Scale

Academic and medical perspectives on ALS focus mostly on the physical aspects of ALS, while psychosocial aspects are accorded secondary importance (McLeod & Clarke, 2007). Individual and caregiver responses to the Functional Rating Scale applied in this study highlight this aspect. More attention needs to be paid to the wider spectrum of the needs of individuals with ALS. This can be achieved by implementing multi-disciplinary approaches, with emphasis on enhancing overall quality of life of the affected individual aside from the physical aspects of the disease.

Over 80% of individuals with ALS experience impairment in verbal communication (Leigh et al., 2003), an ability that was rated by all participants and caregivers in the current study as the most important ability to preserve. Individuals with ALS frequently shift conversations from health-related symptoms to social and relationship issues. This highlights the importance of preserving communication and modifying it according to the individuals' level of communicative ability (Hardiman et al., 2004). AAC strategies used to facilitate communication and address the loss of expressive verbal communication are readily acknowledged within the ALS population (Leigh et al., 2003). However, considerations for the effects of auditory impairment and the associated devices to enhance listening experience are not viewed as equally important. The progression of degeneration gives rise to an increased loss of function and a steady decline in individual day-to-day activity and participation. Hearing loss, be it a direct consequence of ALS or not directly disease-related, poses significant threats to the overall quality of life. When reviewing the effects of disease related symptoms alongside the additional loss of function, such as hearing loss, the increasingly detrimental effects of failing to manage any manageable symptoms on individual quality of life become apparent. This in turn affects the individuals' experience of the disease thereby impacting their ability to manage it (Hardiman et al., 2004; McLeod & Clarke, 2007). The fact that individuals with ALS fail to acknowledge the importance of audition as a key requirement for effective communicative exchange represents a gap in the awareness and management of secondary symptoms in ALS (Hardiman et al., 2004). In contrast, the majority of caregivers in the current study, acknowledged the importance of hearing as a functional skill central to maintaining communicative success. Studies consistently report that significant others are typically more objective in acknowledging the negative effects of hearing impairment and the importance of this on the communicative process (Dalton et al., 2003; Hallam et al., 2008; Starck & Hickson, 2004).

The importance of eating for nutrition to maintain nutritional wellbeing was highlighted by participants in the current study. As individuals' associate deglutition very closely with social success, there is a positive relationship between swallowing success and psychosocial functioning (Ekberg et al., 2002). Participants in the current study alluded to the fact that incompetency in eating is harmful to their individual quality of life, and impact on their ability to maintain individual inclusion in social interactions, which are frequently set around a dining experience. This is supported by the findings of Ekberg et al. (2002) who reported that over 50% of patients with ALS reported eating less throughout the course of the day and found eating to be a displeasurable experience, while 44% of patients reported weight loss within the initial 12 months of symptom presentation.

Arm and leg movement were rated least important in the current study, amongst both individuals with ALS and their caregivers. This suggests that individuals with neurological disease are more readily able to adapt to physical decline by lowering their expectations of physical ability and redirecting this to other areas of life (such as cultural, social and interactive domains). These reports are consistent with Foley et al. (2007) who suggest that the coping strategies implemented by the affected individual reinforces the need for health professionals to consider individuals with ALS beyond their physical disability and in the context of their social and psychological systems.

Communication, hearing, swallowing and vision all contribute to the maintenance of human contact and closeness. Caregivers in the current study viewed hearing as very important. These findings indicate that both individuals with ALS and their caregivers place greater focus on functional abilities (e.g. communication, hearing, swallowing and vision) that would have a direct impact on inclusion and involvement in daily life rather than those abilities related to mobility. Despite increasing disability, individuals with ALS seek to maintain identity, self-worth and respect, of which are achieved through socio-emotional accomplishment (Foley et al., 2007). Although in this study hearing is not equally important for individuals with ALS versus caregivers, the shared notion remains that affected individuals seek to be purposeful, both existentially and socially to maintain psychological wellbeing. In order to achieve this, the primary focus is redirected towards the social and emotional aspects of disease rather than those linked to physical ability (Foley et al., 2007).

Identifying Importance of Auditory Diagnosis

The initial case history interview revealed that the majority of participants in the current study did not report experiencing hearing difficulties, despite auditory testing revealing that they present with hearing loss. This finding is supported by Rawoon and Kiehl (2009) who found that 66.6% of participants in their study had a hearing loss, in contradiction to self-reports suggesting normal hearing. The effects of hearing impairment result in distorted communication, stigmatization and social isolation leading to emotional disturbances as readjustment to the impairment of function is realized (Tambs, 2004). These consequences appear to be highly underestimated by participants in the current study. It has been found that 20.7% of adults with hearing loss seek rehabilitation in the form of hearing aids (Popelka et al., 1998; Rawool & Kiehl, 2009). This indicates that only a small percentage of hearing impaired individuals pursue rehabilitative support, despite research showing that a reduction in depressive symptoms is reported in affected individuals once hearing aid fitting occurs (Tambs, 2004). The decline of these depressive symptoms following the fitting of a hearing aid further highlights the benefits of hearing loss diagnosis and management in individuals with ALS.

The underreporting of hearing loss typically arises as a result of two factors. The first of these may be a result of the individual being unaware of the loss. The severity of communicative difficulties brought about by hearing loss vary according to the severity of the hearing loss, the associated symptoms and the communicative strategies unknowingly implemented to compensate for this (Hallam et al., 2008). Amongst all hearing impaired participants in the current study, hearing loss was isolated to 6000Hz – 8000Hz. A loss in these frequencies tends to impact less on speech recognition abilities in quiet settings. The impact increases though in noisier listening environments and/or as the loss progresses. The majority of the participants in the current study reported that listening experiences in noise proved to be a greater challenge for them. It is therefore likely that hearing loss failed to be acknowledged by individuals as a result of the mild effects of the loss at the time of testing.

As the consequences of motor neuron degeneration extend from a physical level, emotional and social consequences continue to arise. Underreporting of hearing loss may also be linked to denial of auditory disabilities and declining communicative function (Hallam et al., 2008; Hallberg, 2008; Rawool & Kiehl, 2009). Denial is a typical response that protects individuals from stress-provoking situations and serves as an adaptive means to prevent social stigma, and preserve mental integrity and capability (Rawool & Kiehl. 2009). Hallam et al. (2008) support denial as a defense mechanism against accepting hearing loss and suggests that hearing impaired individuals cope with loss through avoiding social situations. Avoidance or minimizing the effects of hearing loss are reported to be more common amongst males than females and occurs as a means of protecting self-image (Garstecki & Erler, 1999; Hallam et al., 2008; Hallberg et al., 2008). This leads to individuals pretending to hear, guessing what was said and/or avoiding interactions. Only 25% of the participants in this study acknowledged experiencing hearing difficulties prior to testing, both of who were female. Interestingly, the male participants in the study who presented with a hearing loss denied the presence of hearing difficulties. This demonstrates the profound psychological burden of ALS in light of the ongoing deterioration of function and the associated experiences of denial linked to new diagnosis. Since hearing loss is invisible it is simpler to deny than the loss of limb function. It is therefore postulated that individuals with ALS may consciously or unconsciously fail to acknowledge hearing difficulties for fear of the negative consequences and the added emotional burden of loss of function beyond the known loss brought about by ALS.

The majority of participants in the current study reported that the knowledge of auditory impairment would be of no importance. Participants approach a diagnosis of hearing loss as an additional negative, untreatable effect. This frame of thought may not be surprising in view of the diagnosis of ALS and its limited rehabilitative opportunities beyond symptom management. It is however suggestive of the need for more active involvement of audiologists in the MDT. This role should include patient education, diagnosis, management and counseling as a means of enhancing patient quality of life. It is postulated individuals who are psychologically isolated and do not believe their symptoms can be helped, will not complain profusely to health professionals in search of alleviation of concerns, but rather become fatalistic about their condition (Ekberg, 2002). Other professionals' lacking the knowledge and understanding of the profound social and psychological effects of hearing impairment, may further negatively impact the early diagnosis and management of hearing loss. Raising health professionals' awareness of the detrimental effects of hearing loss on the quality of life of the individual with ALS, may result in a marked decline in the extent of psychological and social damage that may otherwise arise. Participants in the current study voluntarily remained at the test site for an average of 45 minutes with discussions based on individual auditory symptoms and experiences. This is further testament to the dire need for education, counseling and support related to communication and hearing abilities expressed by these individuals and their caregivers.

The acceptance of hearing loss is directly related to the severity of symptoms (Hogg, Goldstein & Leigh, 1994). These symptoms are often more recognizable to caregivers and surrounding communicative partners, than the hearing impaired individual himself (Hogg et al., 1994). This was evident in the current study, where the majority of caregivers identified auditory diagnosis to be of much greater importance when compared to the individuals with ALS themselves. The severity of functional impairment has a significant relationship to the psychological wellbeing of individuals with ALS, which has marked implications for rehabilitative approaches (Hunter, Robinson & Neilson, 1993). While the severity of functional impairment has been proven to be harmful to psychological wellbeing in neurodegenerative patients, failure to manage symptoms that are to varying extents manageable, further aggravate harmful consequences. The foremost of these consequences is the amplified the levels of distress and emotional anxiety faced by the affected individual. Alongside a gradual progression of hearing impairment, functional and social communicative abilities gradually prove more challenging, leading to experiences of distress and isolation. When failing to address these symptoms, in addition to the less manageable symptoms of ALS, the psychosocial disadvantages are likely to increase. Thus, the ability to manage the presentation of any symptom, whether it is related or unrelated to the disease itself serves to enhance and promote better quality of life for the individual.

It has been found that patients with terminal illness report improved coping resources, closer interpersonal relationships and newly defined life priorities as a result of counseling and understanding symptoms (Averill et al., 2007). In a study conducted by Rawool and Kiehl (2009) it was found that counseling plays an important role in the acceptance of hearing loss. Counseling allows for the exploration of the emotional impact of a diagnosis of hearing impairment and equips the individual with the necessary coping and compensatory strategies as well as amplification necessary to enhance auditory performance. Counseling for hearing loss when viewed in conjunction with the range of difficulties faced by the individual with ALS, is essential as a means of educating and empowering individuals with knowledge of the risks and rehabilitative strategies available to facilitate the difficulties experienced (Hallam et al., 2008). Equipping the individual with this support, knowledge and resources promote improved communicative behaviours which may be implemented by both the caregiver and the hearing impaired individual (Hallberg, 1999). The latter serves to limit the demise of interpersonal relationships on account of hearing impairment, guiding the process of mutual acknowledgment and understanding of the associated burdens faced by all individuals affected by the hearing impairment. This facilitates a recreation of respect for dignity, autonomy and capabilities of the affected individual, while alleviating some burden on both communicative partners (Hallam et al., 2008). This is particularly relevant where the deterioration of speech ability in ALS brings along a different set of obstacles detrimental to the individuals autonomy, involvement and communicative inclusion. It has also been reported by Rawool and Kiehl (2009) that 20% of participants in their study who initially accepted their diagnosis, reverted to their original state of denial of the hearing loss one month after counseling. This further emphasizes the importance of including the audiologist as a permanent member of the multi-disciplinary management team, with their role including the ongoing provision of counseling and support to facilitate individual success at a social level of engagement.

Activities of daily living relate to global functioning activities, including bed-chair mobility or short distance mobility to reach a toilet (UNESCAP, 2008). Although hearing loss cannot be isolated as a direct cause of individual failure to accomplish these goals, impaired hearing ability is firmly acknowledged as an additional element exarbating the levels of difficulty experienced (Dalton et al., 2003). This supports the notion that hearing loss substantially enhances the challenges faced by the individual with ALS when paired alongside general functional decline and the frailty that accompanies disease (Dalton et al., 2003). It is postulated that as the life expectancy of individuals with ALS increases (through medical advances and symptom management), a greater prevalence of hearing impairment will be documented.

Individual differences such as personality and methods of coping are potentially critical for understanding the high variability in disease course (Averill et al., 2007; UNESCAP, 2008). Willingness to remain engaged in daily life, motivation to explore compensatory techniques, devices that accommodate loss of function, positive attitudes and an internal locus of control form essential traits that contribute to living successfully with ALS (Averill et al.,

2007). It has been found that individuals with hearing impairment wait for 5 – 15 years before seeking professional help to improve hearing difficulties (Rawool & Kiehl. 2009). This further highlight the lengthy process involved in acknowledging hearing loss and suggests that this process often exceeds the lifespan of an individual with ALS. It is therefore of upmost importance that ALS management plans emphasize the importance of optimizing functional abilities (such as hearing) that are to a certain extent manageable and that this is done with time urgency. The latter invites positive improvements in quality of life and limits the extent of communicative difficulties faced by the individual with ALS.

Studies suggest that significant others tend to be more objective with regards to acknowledging and reporting the negative impact of hearing loss on communication (Dalton et al., 2003; Hallam et al., 2008; Starck & Hickson, 2004). Evidence of interpersonal stress is reported in 53% of marriages where one individual is affected by hearing loss (Hallam et al., 2008). The impact of hearing impairment on the significant other has been observed to be more severe than that of the individual with the hearing loss (Hallam et al., 2008). This supports the findings of this study whereby caregivers were generally more supportive than the participants with ALS to pursue auditory diagnosis.

The impact of hearing loss on close relationships emphasizes the need for professionals to provide family-based support to facilitate adjustment in contrast to isolated patient-centered support (Hallberg, 1999). Changes in previous communicative patterns and domestic, social and leisure activities require modification in the presence of hearing loss. The mutual willingness of the individual with hearing loss and family members to engage with the problem is paramount (Hallam et al., 2008). This is of particular importance since the stressors experienced by the different parties are often vastly different, creating the opportunity for misunderstanding, conflict and blame. Hogan (2001) report that where a mutual willingnss to accept, acknowledge and manage the presence of hearing loss is not shared, 47.3% of relationships between caregivers and hearing impaired individuals, suffer.

The management of auditory impairment through aural rehabilitation strategies has contributed to improved individual success in existential and social contexts, ultimately enriching individual quality of life (Starck & Hickson, 2004). The psychological benefits of managing new symptoms therefore outweigh the perceived psychological harm of diagnosis, despite the overwhelming rejection of this claim from affected individuals (Rawool & Kiehl. 2009). These benefits cannot however be achieved without establishing a level of equilibrium between perspectives of hearing loss as viewed by both parties.

Conclusion

The involvement of certain pathways and lack of involvement of others plays an important role in the diagnosis of ALS; however prominent sensory symptoms complicate the ease of diagnostic clarity (Pall, 1995). There is a growing body of evidence that suggests the involvement of sensory pathways in ALS. As life-prolonging measures continue to expand lifespan of individuals with ALS, the sensory, autonomic and oculomotor pathways may emerge as more prominent features of ALS than currently accepted (Pall, 1995). The involvement of the auditory pathways when superimposed on the current features of ALS may prove to be catastrophic to the maintenance of individual wellbeing and quality of life.

Furthermore, as the life span of individuals with ALS extends, the possibility of acquiring a presbycutic hearing loss increases. This could be a major factor influencing individual involvement in communicative contexts, whereby the vast adverse effects of hearing loss on social and emotional health lead to a decline in societal and social engagements, withdrawal and loss of autonomy (Rawool & Kiehl, 2009). Where quality of life and the ability to adjust to loss of function are described as the foundation to maintaining individual desire to be socially engaged at a familial and a community level, the additional consequences of sensory effects such as auditory impairment become of critical importance.

In the face of incurable, terminal illness, control over manageable symptoms need to addressed with urgency within the multi-disciplinary management plan. Minimizing the devastating consequences of the disease as a whole and strengthening the involvement and inclusion of the affected individual in day-to-day interactive processes shapes desire to live, which should remain a priority in disease management. Hearing ability affords individuals enhanced quality of experiences in life and considerations for this category of disease management should never be undermined in the management process.

> "I stand alone in a great crowd of ALS 'sufferers', but to be acknowledged and have my opinions respected reminds me that I am still here. I don't know what tomorrow brings, but as long as I am seen I will wake up each morning with more anticipation (than the last) and look forward to the contributions (small or big) that I can make. My body will stop fighting only when my value in the world is abandoned"
>
> Quote from P3

Conclusion

The current research was a preliminary effort to deal with the obvious lack of information on the prevalence of hearing loss in South African individuals diagnosed with adult-onset ALS. A number of limitations were however identified. The limited sample size is one of the primary limitations of the study. Notwithstanding the efforts by the researcher, the unique circumstances of each participant, the unpredictable nature of ALS, and a high attrition rate, only a limited the number of participants could be included in the study. Factors such as locating individuals with ALS representative of the general population and encouraging individual involvement proved challenging. The limited sample size eliminated the researchers' ability to obtain a sample representative of all stages of disease progression, which would have allowed for further analysis into the impact of ALS on the auditory system at the various stages of disease progression. Similarly, the limited sample size further eliminated the ability to review results according to the different types of ALS (spinal, bulbar and mixed). The use of a limited sample size affects statistical analysis procedures linked to achieving confidence intervals of 95% and interpretation of p-values, emphasizing the need for calculated balance in the interpretation of the results (Hackshaw, 2008).

Participants in the more terminal stages of the disease were not included due to the marked deterioration of physical function linked to mobility, speech and respiratory function as well as the fatigue and emotionally taxing demands experienced during this time. This eliminated the researchers' ability to obtain a sample representative of all stages of disease progression, which would have allowed for further analysis into the impact of ALS on the auditory system at the various stages of disease progression.

While the above limitations are critical considerations to hold for future studies, small samples are possibly a more desirable route when examining new research hypothesis, such as in the current study (Hackshaw, 2008). One should consider that the use of a small sample size may not reveal a relationship which would only be exposed when applying the same methodology to a larger sample.

Progressive, neurodegenerative diseases such as ALS often has a negative on the individual on both a level of physical structure and function as well as participation and activities of daily living as described by the ICF framework. All of which have a marked negative impact individual quality of life.

The inclusion of sensory neuropathy as a clinical feature of the ALS spectrum remains a cause of diagnostic uncertainty. However, with recent medical developments and the consequent prolongation of lifespan, the wider spectrum of ALS related signs and symptoms are anticipated to become clinically apparent (Isaacs et al., 2007; Shaw, 2005). Since curative treatments for ALS have yet to be discovered, the challenge in a terminally, progressive disease lies with optimizing individual quality of life. This is largely achieved through maintaining a sense of autonomy and independence – two components that are negatively affected by hearing loss. A loss or decline in auditory function is a key marker associated with declining individual independence and is typically associated with withdrawal and voluntary or involuntary exclusion from social situations, hence threatening individual quality of life.

The management of diseases of a multi-systemic nature, such as ALS, is best met by multi-disciplinary teamwork. Management should focus on symptomatic and rehabilitative measures, encompassing physical and environmental factors that span across the spectrum of ALS (Ng & Khan, 2011). Investigation surrounding the atypical features of ALS is therefore essential for the purpose of refining the standard clinical description of ALS and redefining management plans for each individual. This aims to address and accommodate disease features at both a primary and secondary level as far as medical and rehabilitative management currently allow (Isaacs et al., 2007). This further validates the need for research into less explored domains of ALS - in this instance, auditory function and the associated implications.

Recommendations for Future Research

A number of opportunities for further research surrounding ALS and the auditory system include first and foremost, replicating this study using a larger sample size. Alongside the recruitment of a larger sample size, future research may wish to explore the differences in audiological presentation in the various types of ALS (spinal, bulbar and mixed). In addition, future research may aim to conduct a longitudinal study tracking auditory function across the disease progression. It is further recommended to expand the audiological test battery used in this study to include the assessment of the higher levels of the brainstem and the cortex with measures such as the mid-latency response and the late-latency response. This would further aid auditory testing in this population, by eliminating the requirement for more demanding and physically taxing behavioural test measures and replacing these with less strenuous electrophysiological measures. Qualitative research exploring the understanding of the benefits of audiologists as part of the ALS management team from the perspective of the persons with ALS, their caregivers, audiologists, and the multidisciplinary team involved in the management of the individuals with ALS will also be valuable.

Clinical Implications

The most important clinical implication of the current study is that individuals with ALS are likely to experience hearing loss to various extents and severity during the course of the disease. While it cannot be ascertained with such a limited sample size whether hearing loss is directly related to ALS or natural aging, indicators suggest hearing impairment is likely to pose a threat to communicative success at some stage over the course of the disease.

The majority of current ALS research relates to the physical consequences of motor neuron degeneration. While the significance of these physical symptoms should not be undermined, it is apparent that individuals with ALS shift their focus away from physical abilities and towards maintenance of quality of life, dignity and autonomy. This study exposes the devastating outcome of hearing loss on individual autonomy and interpersonal relationships and highlights the importance of acknowledging the effects this poses on maintaining quality of life despite deterioration of physical ability. This knowledge serves to contribute to the body of information directed at promoting enhanced quality of life for individuals with ALS.

The large variations in the perspectives of individuals with ALS and their caregivers relating to auditory diagnosis emphasize the need for counseling units to equip families to succeed in and maintain quality of life in the presence of hearing impairment. This should be aimed at the immediate family unit as a whole rather than isolated symptomatic management of the affected individual. This support should further be ongoing in nature as opposed to a once off opportunity and would serve to take into account the burden experienced by the caregivers and the individuals with ALS.

As a result the likelihood of hearing impairment and the limited reported involvement of the audiological discipline, this study highlights the need for expansion of the multi-disciplinary ALS team to include the services of the audiological discipline. It is important to also empower individuals with knowledge and understanding of the detrimental effects of hearing impairment. Identifying this gap is of great value for building a body of evidence to promote an increase in audiological counseling and rehabilitative services available to populations in need of multi-disciplinary management.

References

Abe, K. (2000). Cognitive function in amyotrophic lateral sclerosis. *ALS and Other Motor Neuron Disorders, 1,* 343 - 347.

Armero, O.E. (2001). Effects of denied hearing loss on the significant other. *The Hearing Journal, 54* (5), 44-47.

Aronson A., Ramig L., Winholtz W., & Silber S. (1992) Rapid voice tremor or "flutter" in amyotrophic lateral sclerosis. *Annals of Otology, Rhinology and Laryngology, 101*, 511-518.

Averill, A.J., Kasarskis, E.J., & Segerstrom, S.C. (2007). Psychological health in patients with amyotrophic lateral sclerosis. *Amyotrophic Lateral Sclerosis, 8*, 243-254.

Babbi, E., & Mouton, J. (2001). *The practice of social research: South African edition*. Cape Town: Oxford Publishers.

Ball, L.J., Beukelman, D.R., & Pattee, G.L. (2004). Communication effectiveness of individuals with amyotrophic lateral sclerosis. *Journal of Communication Disorders, 37,* 197 - 215.

Bartnik, G., Hawley, M.L., Rogowski, M., Raj-Koziak, D., Fabijanska, A., & Formby, C. (2009). Distortion product otoacoustic emission levels and input/output- growth functions in normal-hearing individuals with tinnitus and/or hyperacusis. *Otolaryngologia Polska, 63*(2), 171-181.

Bess, F.H., & Humes, L.E. (2008). *Audiology: The fundementals* (4th Ed.). Philadelphia: Lippincott Williams and Wilkins.

Block, M.G., & Wiley, T.L. (1994). Overview and basic principles of acoustic immittance measurements. In J. Katz (Ed.), *Handbook of Clinical Audiology (5th Ed.).* (pp. 132-146). Baltimore: Williams & Wilkins.

Brandy, W. (2002). Speech audiometry. In J. Katz (Ed.), *Handbook of Clinical Audiology (5th Ed.).* (pp. 96 – 110). Baltimore: Lippincott Williams & Wilkins.

Brown, J.B., Lattimer, V., & Tudball, T. (2006). An investigation of patients and providers' views of services for motor neuron disease. *British Journal of Neuroscience Nursing, 1* (5), 249-252.

Chia, E.M., Wang, J.J., Rochtchina, E., Cumming, R.R., Newall, P., & Mitchell, P. (2007). Hearing impairment and health related quality of life: The Blue Mountains hearing study. *Ear and Hearing, 28,* 187-195.

Clark, J.L., Roeser, R.J., & Mendrygal, M. (2007). Middle Ear Measures. In R.J. Roeser,M. Valente, & H. Hosford-Dunn (Eds.), *Auditory Diagnosis,* (pp. 380-389). New York: Thieme Medical Publishers.

Dalton, D.S., Cruickshanks, K.J., Klein, B.E.K., Klein, R., Wiley, T.L., & Nondahl, D.M. (2002). The impact of hearing loss on quality of life in older adults. *The Gerontologist, 43*(5), 661-668.

Dewane, C. (2010). Hearing loss in older adults – its effects on mental health. *Social Work Today, 10*(4), 18-21.

Dirks, D.D (2002). Bone Conduction. In J. Katz (Ed.), *Handbook of Clinical Audiology* (pp. 132-146). Baltimore: Lippincott Williams & Wilkins.

Don, M., & Kwong, B. (2002). Auditory brainstem response: Differential diagnosis. In J. Katz (Ed.), *Handbook of Clinical Audiology* (5th Ed.). (pp. 274-297). Baltimore: Lippincott Williams & Wilkins.

Donaghy, M. (1999). Classification and clinical features of motor neurone diseases and motor neuropathies in adults. *Journal of Neurology, 246,* 331 - 333.

Donaghy, C., Dick, A., Hardiman, O., & Patterson, V. (2008). Timeliness of diagnosis in motor neurone disease: A population-based study. *Ulster Medical Journal, 77*(1), 18- 21.

Doyle, M., & Phillips, B. (2001). Trends in AAC use by individuals with ALS. *Augmentative and Alternative Communication, 17*(3), 167-178.

Duffy, J.R. (2005). *Motor speech disorders: Substrates, Differential diagnosis and management* (2nd Ed.). London: Elsevier Mosby, Inc.

Ekberg, O., Hamdy, S., Woisard, V., Wuttge-Hannig, A., & Ortega, P. (2002). Social and psychological burden of dysphagia: Its impact on diagnosis and treatment. *Dysphagia, 11*, 139 – 146.

Erber, N.P., & Scherer, S.C (1999). Sensory loss and communication difficulties in the elderly. *Australasian Journal on Aging, 18*(1), 4-9.

Erdman, S.A. (2009). The need for a new medical model: A challenge for biomedicine. *Science, 296*, 129-136.

Foley. G., O'Mahony, P., & Hardiman, O. (2007). Perceptions of quality of life in people with ALS: Effects of coping and health care. *Amyotrophic Lateral Sclerosis, 8*, 164- 169.

Freed, D. (2000). *Motor speech disorders: Diagnosis and treatment*. San Diego: Singular Publishing.

Gagne, J.P., Jennings, M.B., & Southall, K (2009). The international classification of functioning: Implications and applications to audiologic rehabilitation. In J.J. Motano, & J.B. Spitzer (Eds.), *Adult Audiologic Rehabilitation* (pp. 37-61). San Diego, California: Plural Publishers.

Garstecki, D.C., & Erler, S.F. (1999). Older adult performance on the communication profile for the hearing impaired. *Journal of Speech, Language and Hearing Research*, *42*, 785 - 796.

Gates, G.A., & Mills, J.H. (2005). Presbycusis. *The Lancet, 366*(9491), 1111-1120.

Gelfand, S.A. (2009). *Essentials in audiology (3rd Ed.)*. Baltimore: Lippincott Williams & Wilkins.

Ghadiali, S.N., Swarts, J.D., & Doyle, W.J. (2003). Effect of tensor veli palatini muscle paralysis on eustachian tube mechanics. *The Annals of Otology, Rhinology and Laryngology, 112*, 704 –711.

Glennen, S.L., & DeCoste, D.C. (1997). *The handbook of augmentative and alternative communication*. San Diego: Singular Publishing Group, Inc.

Goldstein, L.H., & Leigh, P.N. (1999). Motor neurone disease: A Review of its emotional and cognitive consequences for patients and its impact on carers. *British Journal of Health Psychology*, *4*(3), 193-208.

Goldstein, L.H., Atkins, L., Landau, S., Brown, R.G., & Leigh, P.N. (2006). Longitudinal predictors of psychological distress and self-esteem in people with ALS. *Neurology*, *67*, 1654 – 1658.

Gorga, M.P., Neely, S.T., Dorn, P.A., & Hoover, B.M (2003). Further efforts to predict pure-tone thresholds from distortion product otoacoustic emission input/output functions. *Acoustical Society of America*, *113*(6), 3275 – 3284.

Gourie-Devi, M., & Suresh, T.G. (1988) Madras Pattern of motor neuron disease in South India. *Journal of Neurology, Neurosurgery and Psychiatry, 51*, 773-777.

Grauman, K., Betke, M., Gips, J., & Bradski, G.R. (2001). Communication via eye blinks: Detection and duration analysis in real time. *IEEE Computer Society Conference on Computer Vision and Pattern Recognition, 1*, 1010.

Hall, J.W., & Mueller, H.G. (1997). *Audiologists desk reference: Volume I Diagnostic audiology principles, procedures and practices*. San Diego: Singular Publishing Group.

Hallam, R., Ashton, P., Sherbourne, K., & Gailey, L. (2008). Persons with acquired profound hearing loss (APHL): How do they and their families adapt to the challenge? *Health: An*

Interdisciplinary Journal for the Social Study of Health, Illness and Medicine, 12 (3), 369-388.

Hallberg, L.R.M. (1999). Hearing impairment, coping and consequences on family life. *Journal of the Academy of Rehabilitative Audiology, 32*, 45-59.

Hallberg, L.R.M., & Barrenas, M.L. (1995). Coping with noise- induced hearing loss: Experiences from the perspective of middle-aged male victims. *British Journal of Audiology, 29*(4), 219 – 230.

Hallberg, L.R.M., Hallberg, U., & Kramer, S.E. (2008). Self-reported hearing difficulties, communication strategies and psychological general wellbeing (quality of life) in patients with acquired hearing impairment. *Disability and Rehabilitation, 30*(3), 203- 212.

Hardiman, O., Hickey, A., & O'Donerty, L.J. (2004) Physical decline and quality of life in Amyotrophic Lateral Sclerosis. *ALS and Other Motor Neuron Disorders, 5*, 230 – 234.

Harrell, R.W. (2002). Pure tone evaluation. In J. Katz (Ed.*), Handbook of Clinical Audiology (5th Ed.).* (pp. 71 – 87). Baltimore: Lippincott Williams & Wilkins.

Hogan, A. (2001). *Hearing rehabilitation for deafened adults: A psychosocial approach.* London: Whurr Publishers.

Hogg, K.E., Goldstein, L.H., & Leigh, P.N. (1994). The psychological impact of motor neurone disease. *Psychological Medicine, 24*, 625-632.

Hunter, M.D., Robinson, I.C., & Neilson, S. (1993). The functional and psychological status of patients with amyotrophic lateral sclerosis: Some implications for rehabilitation. *Disability and Rehabilitation, 15*(3), 119-126.

Isaacs, J.D., Dean, A.F., Shaw, C.E., Al-Chalabi, A., Mills, K.R., & Leigh, P.N. (2007). Amyotrophic lateral sclerosis with sensory neuropathy: part of a multisystem disorder? *Journal of Neurology, Neurosurgery and Psychiatry, 78*, 750-753.

Kelly, B., Burnett, P., Pelusi, D., Badger, S., Varghese, F., & Robertson, M. (2003). Factors associated with the wish to hasten death: A study of patients with terminal illness. *Psychological Medicine, 33,* 75-81.

Kubler, A., Winter, S., Ludolph, M.A., & Birbaumer, N. (2005). Severity of depressive symptoms and quality of life in patients with amyotrophic lateral sclerosis. *Neurorehabilitation and Neural Repair, 19*, 182 – 193.

Kramer, S. (2008). Hearing Impairment, word and vocational enablement. *International Journal of Audiology, 47*(2), 124 – 130.

Kuhnlein, P., Gdynia, H.J., Sperfeld, A.D., Linder-Pfleghar, B., Ludolph, A.C., Prosiegel, M., & Riecker, A. (2008). Nature clinical practice neurology. Diagnosis and treatment of bulbar symptoms in ALS. *Amyotrophic Lateral Sclerosis, 4,* 366 - 374.

Lasker, J. P., & Bedrosian, J. L. (2000). Acceptance of AAC by adults with acquired disorders. In D.R. Beukelman, K.M. Yorkston, & J. Reichle (Eds.), *Augmentative and alternative communication for adults with acquired neurologic disorders* (pp. 107-136). Baltimore: Paul H. Brookes.

Leigh, P.N., Abrahams, S., Al-Chalabi, A., Ampong, M.A., Goldstein, L.H., Johnson, J., … Willey, E. (2003). The management of motor neuron disease. *Journal of Neurology, Neurosurgery and Psychiatry. 74,* 432 - 447.

Logroscino, G., Traynor, B.J., Hardiman, O., Chio, A., Mitchell, D., Swingler, R.J., & Beghi, E. (2008). Descriptive epidemiology of amyotrophic lateral sclerosis: New evidence and unsolved issues. *Journal of Neurology, Neurosurgery & Psychiatry with Practical Neurology, 79*, 6-11.

Maier, A., Linke, P., Dullinger, J., Borisow, N., Munch, C., Bottcher, T & Meyer, T. (2009). Hypoacusis in ALS patients receiving long-term ventilation. *Amyotrophic Lateral Sclerosis, 10*(1), 189.

Marieb, E.N. (2001). *Human anatomy and physiology*. New York. Pearson Education, Inc.

Mathers, C.D., Smith, A., & Concha, M. (2003). *Global burden of hearing loss in the year 2000*. Geneva, World Health Organization.

McLeod, J.E., & Clarke, D.M. (2007). A review of psychosocial aspects of motor neurone disease. *Journal of the Neurological Sciences, 258*, 4 – 10.

Michaud, L., Burnand, B., & Stiefel, F. (2004). Taking care of the terminally ill cancer patient: Delerium as a symptom of terminal disease. *Annals of Oncology, 15*(4), iv199-iv203.

Mitsumoto, H., & Del Bene, M. (2000). Improving the quality of life for people with ALS: The challenge ahead. *ALS and other motor neuron disorders*, *1*(5), 329 – 336.

Mondelli, M., Rossi, A., Passero, S., & Guazzi, G.C. (1993). Involvement of peripheral sensory fibers in amyotrophic lateral sclerosis: Electrophysiological study of 64 cases. *Muscle Nerve, 16*, 166-172.

Murphy, J. (2004). "I prefer contact this close": Perceptions of AAC by people with motor neuron disease and their communication partners. *Augmentative and Alternative Communication, 20*(4), 259-271.

Musiek, F.E., & Baran, J.A. (2007). *The auditory system: Anatomy, Physiology and clinical correlations*. Boston: Allyn and Bacon.

Nachtegaal, J., Smit, J.H., Smits, C., Bezemer, P.D., van Beek, J.H.M., Festen, J.M., & Kramer, S.E. (2009). The association between hearing status and psychosocial health before the age of 70 years: Results from an Internet-Based National Survey. *Ear and Hearing, 30*(3), 302 – 312.

Newman, C.W., Weinstein, B.E., Jacobson, G.P., & Hug, G.A. (1990). The hearing handicap inventory for adults: Psychometric adequacy and audiometric correlates. *Ear and Hearing, 11(6,)* 430-433.

Ng, L., & Khan, F. (2011). Identification of Personal Factors in Motor Neurone Disease: A pilot study. *Rehabilitation Research and Practice*, Article ID 871237, 7 pages, doi:10.1155/2011/871237.

Pall, H.S. (1995). Motor Neuron Disease. *Reviews in Clinical Gerontology, 5*(3), 303 – 311.

Popelka M.M, Cruickshanks K.J., Wiley T.L., Tweed T.S., Klein B.E.K., & Klein R. (1998). Low prevalence of hearing aid use among older adults with hearing loss: The epidemiology of hearing loss study. *Journal of the American Geriatric Society*, *46*(9), 1075-1078.

Pugdahl, K., Fuglsang-Frederiksen, A., de Carvalho, M., Johnsen, B., Fawcett, P.R.W., Labarre-Vila, A., … Schofield, I.S. (2007). Generalised sensory system abnormalities in amyotrophic lateral sclerosis: A European multicentre study. *Journal of Neurology, Neurosurgery, Psychiatry, 78*, 746-749.

Prieve, B.A. & Fitzgerald, T.S. (2002). Otoacoustic Emissions. In J. Katz (Ed.), *Handbook of Clinical Audiology (5th Ed.)*. (pp. 440 - 468). Baltimore: Lippincott Williams & Wilkins.

Rappaport, J.M. & Provencal, C. (2002). Neuro-otology for audiologists. In J. Katz (Ed.), *Handbook of Clinical Audiology (5th Ed.)*. (pp. 9 - 32). Baltimore: Williams & Wilkins.

Rawool, V.W., & Kiehl, J.M. (2009). *Effectiveness of informational counseling on acceptance of hearing loss among older adults.* Hearing Review, http://www.hearingreview.com/issues/articles/2009-06_01.asp

Riviere, M., Meininger, V., Zeisser, P., & Munsat, T. (1998). An Analysis of extended survival in patients with amyotrophic lateral sclerosis treated with riluzole. *Archives of Neurology, 55*, 526 - 528.

Ross, E., & Deverell, A. (2004). *Psychosocial Approached to Health, Illness and Disability: A Reader for health care professionals.* Pretoria: Van Schaiks Publishers.

Royal College of Speech-Language Therapists (2007). Resource manual for commissioning and planning services for speech language and communication needs. Retrieved from Royal College of Speech-Language Therapists website: http://www.rcslt.org/speech_and_language_therapy/commissioning/intro

Schiavetti, N., & Metz, D.E. (2002). *Evaluating Research In Communicative Disorders.* (4th Ed.). Boston: Allyn and Bacon.

Sharp, J.F., Wilson, J.A., Ross, L., & Barr-Hamilton, R.M. (1990). Ear wax removal: A survey of current practices. *British Medical Journal, 301*, 1251-1252.

Shaw, P.J. (2005). Molecular and cellular pathways of neurodegeneration in motor neuron disease. *Journal of Neurology, Neurosurgery and Psychiatry, 76,* 1046 - 1057.

Silverman, D. (2000). *Doing qualitative research: A practical handbook.* California: Sage Publications.

Simmons, Z., Bremer, B.A., Robbins, R.A., Walsh, S.M., & Fischer, S. (2000). Quality of life in ALS depends on factors other than strength and physical function. *Neurology, 55* (3), 388-392.

Snell, R.S. (2001). *Clinical neuroanatomy for medical students.* Philadelphia. Lippincott Williams & Wilkins.

Spoendlin, H. (1971). Degeneration behaviour of the cochlear nerve. *European Archives of Oto-Rhino-Layngology, 200*(4), 275-291.

Spoendlin, H., & Schrott, A. (1989). Analysis of the human auditory nerve. *Hearing Research, 43*(1), 25 – 38.

StatSoft, Inc. (2005). STATISTICA (data analysis software system), version 7.1. www.statsoft.com.

Tambs, K. (2004). Moderate effects of hearing loss on mental health and subjective wellbeing: Results from the Nord Trondelag hearing loss study. *Psychosomatic Medicine, 66*, 776-782.

Tambs, K., Hoffman, H.J., Engdahl, B., & Borchgrevink, H.M. (2004). Hearing loss associated with ear infections in Nord-Trondelag, Norway. *Ear and Hearing, 25*(4), 388-396.

Teijlingen van, E., Rennie, A.M., Hundley, V., & Graham, W. (2001). The importance of conducting and reporting pilot studies: The Example of the Scottish British survey. *Journal of Advanced Nursing, 34*, 289 - 295.

Tesch-Romer, C. (1997). Psychological effects of hearing aid use in older adults. *The Journals of Gerontology, 52*(3), 127-138.

Theys, P.A., Peeters. E., & Robberecht, W. (1999). Evolution of motor and sensory deficits in amyotrophic lateral sclerosis estimated by neurophysiological techniques. *Journal of Neurology, 246*, 438-442.

Thibodeau, L.M. (2007). Speech Audiometry. In R. Roeser,M. Valente, & H. Hosford-Dunn(Eds.) *Audiology: Diagnosis (2nd Ed.).* (pp. 288 – 313). New York: Thieme Medical Publishers.

Traynor, B.J., Codd, M.B., Corr, B., Forde, C., Frost, E., & Hardiman, O.M. (2000). Clinical features of amyotrophic lateral sclerosis according to the El Escorial and Airlie House Diagnostic Criteria. *Archives of Neurology, 57,* 1171 - 1179.

United Nations Economic and Social Commission for Asia and the Pacific. (2004). *First Workshop for Improving Disability Statistics and Measurement Bangkok 24-28 May.* Retrieved from http://www. unescap.org/stat/meet/widsm1/widsm1_nenad2.asp.

Van Damme, P., & Robberecht, W. (2009). Recent advances in motor neuron disease. *Current Opinions in Neurology, 22*, 486 – 492.

Vernon, J.A. (2002). Hyperacusis: Testing, treatments and a possible mechanism. *The Australian and New Zealand Journal of Audiology*, *24*(2), 68 – 73.

Vesterager, V. (1997). Clinical Review: Tinnitus-Investigation and Management. *British Medical Journal*, 314, 728 – 731.

Ward, C.D., Phillips, M., Smith, A., & Moran, M. (2003). Multidisciplinary approached in progressive neurological disease: Can we do better? *Journal of Neurology,Neurosurgery & Psychiatry*, *74*, 8-12.

Weinstein, B.E. (2002). Hearing loss in the elderly: A new look at an old problem. In. J. Katz (Ed.) *Handbook of Clinical Audiology (5th Ed.).* (pp. 597- 606). Baltimore: Williams & Wilkins.

Wijesekera, L.C., & Leigh, P.N. (2009). Amyotrophic Lateral Sclerosis. *Journal of Neurology, Neurosurgery and Psychiatry, 78,* 750 -753.

World Health Organization. (2001). *International Classification of Functioning, Disability and Health.* Geneva, Switzerland, Word Health Organization.

World Health Organization & United Nations Economic and Social Commission for Asia and the Pacific. (2008). *Training Manual on Disability Statistics*, United Nations, Bangkok.

Yorkston, K.M., Beukelman, D.R., Strand, E.A., & Bell, K.R. (1999). *Management in motor speech disorders in children and adults* (2nd Ed.). Austin: Pro-Ed.

Yueh, B., Shapiro, N., MacLean, C.H., & Shekelle, P.G. (2003). Screening and management of adult hearing loss in primary care. *Journal of the American Medical Association, 289,* 1976 - 1985.

In: Amyotrophic Lateral Sclerosis
Editors: Katashi Segawa and Ryota Ijichi

ISBN: 978-1-62257-679-1

Chapter 2

Role of Lipid Transcription Factor, Sterol Regulatory Element Binding Protein 1 (SREBP1) in ALS: Potential Therapeutic Interventions

Siavash Khalaj and Changiz Taghibiglou*
Department of Pharmacology, College of Medicine,
University of Saskatchewan, Saskatoon, Canada

Abstract

Amyotrophic Lateral Sclerosis (ALS) is a progressive neurodegenerative disease which leads to disability and death. A number of potential mechanisms for the development of ALS have been proposed. Emerging evidence strongly suggests a connection between lipid metabolism abnormalities and ALS. Glutamate excitotoxicity has been also identified as one of the major contributing factors mediating cell death in ALS. We have recently established a causative link between glutamate excitotoxicity-induced lipid transcription factor sterol regulatory element binding protein-1 (SREBP1) activation and neuronal apoptosis in ischemic stroke. The inhibition of neuronal SREBP1 by high exogenous cholesterol or a TAT-fused short peptide (Indip) significantly protected neurons both in vitro and in vivo. More recently, we detected a high level of SREBP1 activation in the spinal cord tissues of the G93A mouse model of ALS and post-mortem ALS patients indicating a pivotal role for the lipid transcription factor in the pathogenesis of ALS. In this chapter, we will discuss our findings on NMDA subtype glutamate receptor overexcitation induced SREBP1 activation and neuronal apoptosis as well as potential therapeutic benefits of modulating this lipid transcription signaling pathway in ALS treatment.

Keywords: ALS, Excitotoxicity, NMDAR, SREBP1, Lipid, Indip, Neuroprotection

* Corresponding Author: Dr. Changiz Taghibiglou, Department of Pharmacology, College of Medicine, 107 Wiggins Road, Health Sciences Bldge. Saskatoon, SK, S7N 5E5, Canada; changiz.taghibiglou@usask.ca.

INTRODUCTION

Amyotrophic Lateral Sclerosis (ALS) or Lou Gehrig's disease is an adult-onset fatal neurodegenerative disease characterized by progressive apoptosis of upper and lower motor neurons in the brain, brainstem and spinal cord. This results in paralysis of bulbar, limb, thoracic and abdominal skeletal muscles, and death within 2–5 years of diagnosis [1]. Respiratory failure, aspiration pneumonia caused by dysphagia and pulmonary embolisms following prolonged immobility are the causes of death.

ALS is a rare disease with an incidence of approximately 2 per 100,000 per year in Western countries, with a higher incidence among men (3.0 per 100,000 per year) than among women (2.4 per 100,000 per year) [2]. It is estimated that the overall lifetime risk of developing ALS is 1:400.

Approximately 5% of ALS patients inherit the disease in an autosomal dominant fashion (familial ALS or FALS) [3], whereas the majority of ALS patients (~ 95%) have no apparent genetic linkage (sporadic ALS or SALS) (reviewed in [4, 5]). While SALS appears to occur with a higher incidence in males compared to females, FALS has a similar incidence in both genders.

Almost 15-20% of familial ALS cases are associated with a mutation in the copper/zinc ion-binding superoxide dismutase type 1 (SOD1) gene [6-8]. SOD1 is a ubiquitously expressed free radical scavenger that reduces cellular oxidative stress by catalyzing the conversion of superoxide anions to hydrogen peroxide and molecular oxygen (Reviewed in [9]). More than hundred mutations in the SOD1 gene have been identified in FALS. Although oxidative stress plays an important role in cellular death, the mechanisms by which these mutations in SOD1 result in apoptosis in motor neurons of ALS patients have not yet been fully understood [10]. There is strong evidence indicating that the toxicity of mutant SOD1 in ALS is most likely due to SOD1 gaining toxic functions rather than losing enzymatic activity [10]. It is believed that mutant SOD1 stimulates oxidative stress and induces mitochondrial dysfunction, excitotoxicity, inflammation, and protein aggregation. Dominant mutations in the genes encoding two highly structurally and functionally similar DNA/RNA binding proteins that harbor prion-like domains, TDP-43 (TAR DNA binding protein) and FUS/TLS (fusion in sarcoma/translated in liposarcoma) are also attributed to the pathogenesis of FALS [11-14]. Both FUS and TDP-43 play important roles in DNA transcription and RNA processing since they shuttle between the nucleus and cytoplasm. Each of these mutated genes contributes to 5% of FALS cases. Moreover, both of these proteins have been identified as components of pathological ubiquitinated inclusions in neurons of ALS patients [15, 16]. Mutations of TAF15, another RNA binding protein with prion-like domain has also been identified in postmortem spinal cord of ALS patients [17].Most recently, Deng et al. have linked mutations in the UBQLN2 gene which encodes the ubiquitin-like protein ubiquilin-2 to dominant X-linked juvenile and adult-onset ALS and ALS/dementia [18]. There are less frequent mutated genes identified in FALS cases such as in the gene encoding VAMP (vesicle associated membrane protein) associated protein B(VAPB) [19, 20], mutations in the ANG (angiogenin), a hypoxia responsive gene [21], and mutations in the gene encoding optineurin (OPTN), which is a causative gene of primary open-angle glaucoma (POAG) [22]. These gene mutations account for about 30-35% of all FALS cases. More genome-wide association studies are required to identify still unknown genetic mutations involved in the pathogenesis of familial ALS. The cause of the remaining 90-95% of patients diagnosed with ALS and classified as sporadic ALS patients is largely unknown. ALS is considered a multifactorial disease with multiple pathophysiological mechanisms resulting from complex environmental interactions with genetic and molecular pathways [23-25]. In terms of environmental risk factors, a variety of factors have been proposed, such as individual's previous engagement in professional sports or intensive physical activities [26-28], serving in the US armed forces [29,30], tobacco and cigarette smoking [31-33], and exposure to neurotoxins [34-37].

At the cellular and molecular levels, compelling evidence indicates that as the disease starts and progresses, neurons undergo drastic alterations such as increased oxidative stress [10], compromised mitochondrial functions (recently reviewed in [38-40]), changes in glutamate receptors function and signaling, increased neuronal excitability, impaired protein ubiquitination (reviewed in [41]) and endoplasmic reticulum (ER) stress (reviewed in [42]), impaired axonal transport (reviewed in [43]), astrocytes and glial dysfunction (reviewed in [44, 45]), and impaired Ca^{2+} buffering [46] leading to neuronal loss and apoptosis.

Several studies have also implicated different transcription factors such as SP1 [47], Nrf2 [48], PPARγ [49], P53 [50], ATF3 [51], c-Jun [52], HoXB2 [53], HSF-1 [54], CREB [55], NF-kB [56,57], CCAAT/enhancer binding protein β (C/EBPβ) [58], and Hypoxia inducible factor-1 (HIF-1) (reviewed in [59]) in the pathogenesis of ALS. Using cultured rat cortical and hippocampal neurons as well as MCAO (middle cerebral artery occlusion) as an in vivo model of stroke, we established a direct causative link between neuronal excitotoxicity-induced activation of the lipogenic transcription factor sterol regulatory element binding protein-1 (SREBP1) and neuronal cell death (Figure 1) [60].

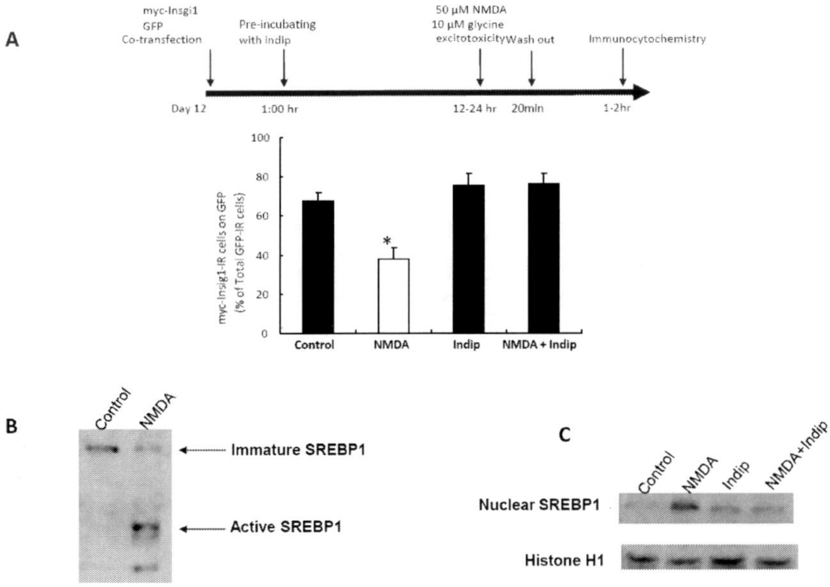

Figure 1. Indip stabilizes Insig-1 and reduces NMDA-dependent SREBP-1 activation. (A) Analysis of immunocytochemistry data for Myc-Insig-1 degradation after NMDA insult in the presence and absence of Indip. n=5, * p<0.001, * P<0.001 (One Way ANOVA), error bar=S.E.M. (B) Activation of SREBP1 in cultured cortical neurons 6 h post NMDA excitotoxic insult (total lysate). (C) Nuclear SREBP-1 immunoblot 6 h after excitotoxic NMDA insult in the presence of Indip.

Most recently, we detected activation of SREBP1 in the G93A mouse model of ALS and postmortem human spinal cord samples indicating an important role for the excitotoxicity-induced activation of the lipid transcription factor in the pathogenesis of ALS [61].

ALS is associated with impaired energy homeostasis and metabolism including hypermetabolism and dyslipidemia, as well as weight loss. Increasing reports from both animal and human studies suggest the involvement of lipid metabolism and energy homeostasis in the progression and outcome of ALS. There is a negative correlation between impaired energy metabolism and progression of the disease (reviewed in [62]). In fact, the nutritional status of patients is one of the important factors determining the survival time period in ALS, besides important factors such as clinical presentation at the time of diagnosis, rate of disease progression, and early presence of respiratory failure [5]. A better understanding of molecular and cellular mechanisms involved in the pathogenesis of ALS will assist in introducing new therapeutic measures to extend life expectancy and improve the quality of life in ALS patients.

In this review, we discuss the contribution of excitotoxicity, particularly NMDA receptor dependent overexcitation and activation of SREBP1 in motor neuron death, and propose a mechanism to connect this novel deleterious signaling pathway to the beneficial effects of high fat diet and Indip, a SREBP1 inhibitory short peptide in ALS.

The Role of Excitotoxicity in the Pathogenesis of ALS

At glutamatergic synapses, glutamate release from the presynaptic neuronal terminals activates ionotropic glutamate receptors at the postsynaptic site. Activation of these receptors allows the influx of Ca^{2+} and Na^{+} (second messengers) leading to neuronal membrane depolarization and generation of action potentials. The action of glutamate is terminated by its rapid uptake from the synaptic cleft by glutamate transporters present in neurons and astrocytes, particularly by the high affinity EAAT2/GLT-1 transporters on astrocyte plasma membranes. The excitatory amino acid transporter-2 (EAAT2), also called glutamate transporter-1 (GLT-1) is primarily expressed on astrocytes as well as neurons and oligodendrocytes throughout the brain and spinal cord. EAAT2 is responsible for more than 90% of glutamate uptake [63, 64]. In pathological conditions, extracellular glutamate concentrations are increased to non-physiologic and toxic levels (~2-5 μM) due to excessive presynaptic release and/or insufficiency in glutamate re-uptake process by glutamate transporters [65]. Moreover, glutamate released from weakened and dying neurons also contributes to the elevation of this excitatory amino acid in the synaptic cleft and its vicinity (reviewed in [66]). Excessive extracellular glutamate levels over-stimulate or overexcite glutamate receptors causing massive Ca^{2+} and Na^{+} influx and activation of calcium-dependent deleterious intracellular signaling pathways, which lead to neuronal death. This phenomenon is called excitotoxicity. Although glutamate-induced neuronal toxicity was reported and characterized in retinal and spinal neurons more than 50 years ago [67, 68], the term "excitotoxicity" was coined by Choi about 30 years later [69]. Glutamate-induced excitotoxicity is involved in the pathogenesis of stroke, trauma, epilepsy and neurodegenerative diseases such as Alzheimer's disease, Parkinson's disease, Huntington's disease and ALS [66, 70-74].

As mentioned earlier, the pathogenesis of ALS is complicated, multifactorial and still unclear. In addition to glutamate excitotoxicity, other important factors including genetics, oxidative stress, hypoxia, mitochondrial abnormalities, impaired neurotrophic support, axonal transport disruption, altered glial function, dysfunction of the Na^{+}/K^{+} ion pump, neurofilament disorganization, autophagy, proteasome dysfunction, viral infection, immune imbalance and compromised functions of the blood-brain, blood-spinal cord and blood-cerebrospinal fluid barriers have been implicated in the pathogenesis of ALS. Here, we will only discuss the role of glutamate-induced excitotoxicity in the pathogenesis of ALS, whereas, other equally important factors have been comprehensively reviewed elsewhere [43, 62, 75].

The detection of relatively high levels of glutamate in the CSF (cerebral spinal fluid) samples of ALS patients compared to age and gender matched healthy subjects provides evidence for the involvement of excitotoxicity in ALS [76-79]. Although this observation has been challenged [80], however, it is supported by reports indicating a significant selective loss of GLT-1 in the post-mortem spinal cord and motor cortex specimens of ALS patients [81, 82] as well as mouse models of ALS [83-85]. Furthermore, reducing excitatory inputs has been proven to be neuroprotective by delaying the onset of disease in the SOD1 mouse model of ALS [86, 87]. More evidence for the role of glutamatergic toxicity in ALS came from the observation of neuroprotection after blocking of ionotropic glutamate receptors *in vitro* using AMPAR and NMDAR antagonists [88, 89], as well as detection of gradual selective motor neuron death following the intrathecal injection of the glutamate agonist kainic acid in normal rat [87]. The perfusion of AMPA in the rat lumbar spinal cord also caused remarkable loss of spinal motor neurons and produced ALS-like symptoms, which were prevented by an AMPAR antagonist, indicating a pivotal role for AMPARs in the pathogenesis of ALS [90].

Among the glutamate receptors, the role of AMPAR-dependent excitotoxicity has been extensively studied in ALS (reviewed in [66, 75, 91]). AMPARs are tetrameric assemblies of highly homologous subunits encoded by four different genes, GluA1-4 (also known as GluR1-4) which mediate fast excitatory synaptic transmission in the mammalian brain (recently reviewed in [92]). The presence of the GluA2 (GluR2) subunit in AMPAR assemblies determines their Ca^{2+} permeability, since GluA2 is almost Ca^{2+} impermeable. The mRNA of GluA2 is subjected to post-transcriptional editing by the adenosine deaminase acting on RNA type 2 enzyme (ADAR2), which converts a key glutamine codon (Gln;Q) at the channel entry (aa at the 607 position) to a codon for arginine (Arg;R). The positively charged arginine prevents Ca^{2+} influx in the GluA2-containing AMPARs (Reviewed in [93]). Those AMPARs lacking the GluA2 subunit or containing the unedited version of it (GluA2Q) remain highly Ca^{2+} and Na^{+} permeable in contrast to the low Ca^{2+} conductance of those containing the edited form of the GluA2 subunit. The abundance of unedited GluA2 (GluA2Q) containing AMPARs in the CNS is less than 1%. The expression levels of GluA2Q (unedited)-containing AMPARs increases in pathological CNS conditions such as ischemia [94], epilepsy [95, 96], glioblastoma progression [97, 98] and ALS [99, 100].

Kawahara et al. demonstrated that GluA2 subunit mRNA editing was defective in the spinal motor neurons of 56% of individuals affected by ALS [99]. Therefore, inefficient and defective ADAR2 enzymatic function resulting in abnormal motor neuron AMPAR expression profile in ALS patients may contribute to their vulnerability to AMPAR-mediated excitotoxicity and motor neuron death. The AMPAR subunit alteration has also been reported in motor neurons of G93A mouse model of ALS [101].

Furthermore, the lumbar co-perfusion of AMPA with either a selective blocker of GluA2-lacking AMPARs (1-naphtyl acetyl spermine), or an intracellular calcium ion chelator effectively and equally prevented motor neuron damage and paralysis in rat, indicating the deleterious role of GluA2-lacking calcium permeable AMPA receptor overexcitation in the spinal cord motor neurons in ALS [102].

Moreover, abnormal control of motor neuronal excitability through an imbalance between excitatory glutamate/D-serine and inhibitory glycine/γ-amino butanoic acid (GABA) neuronal functions may also contribute to the excitotoxicity-induced neurodegeneration in ALS (reviewed by [103]).

The role of *N*-methyl-d-aspartate receptors (NMDARs) in the pathogenesis of ALS has not been thoroughly investigated. NMDA sensitive glutamate receptors are highly Ca^{2+} permeable, heterotetrameric ligand-gated ion channels composed of the obligatory GluN1 (NR1) subunit with at least one type of GluN2 (NR2) (GluN2A to D) and/or GluN3 subunits. The majority of NMDARs in the CNS contain GluN2B (NR2B) or GluN2A (NR2A) subunits. Different GluN2 subunits produce different downstream signaling and have distinct electrophysiological and pharmacological properties, which couples them with different signaling machineries. Thus, the activation of NMDARs may have different functional consequences based on the GluN2A and GluN2B-containing NMDAR subpopulations [104-106]. The occupation of the co-agonist binding site on the NMDAR is required for its activation by glutamate. In the mammalian brain, D-serine is a physiological ligand of the co-agonist site of the NMDARs [107]. The NMDARs present in the CNS are essential for brain development and play key physiological roles in neuronal survival, and functions [108-110]. However, overstimulation of NMDARs, particularly those containing the GluN2B subunit, causes neuronal excitotoxicity due to the accumulation of excessive intraneuronal Ca^{2+} and incomplete desensitization. This contributes to neuronal death in ischemia, hypoxia [74, 111], and in chronic neurodegenerative diseases [112-114]. Paradoxically, the activation of GluN2A containing NMDARs promotes neuronal survival [115, 116]. It appears that the precise localization of NMDARs (synaptic vs. extrasynaptic), as well as their subunit composition, determines the physiological/pathological outcomes following their overactivation [4, 71, 72, 105, 117]. It is noteworthy that the expression of GluN2A, the neuroprotective subunit of NMDAR, is significantly decreased in both dorsal and ventral horns of post-mortem spinal cords of ALS patients compared with control subjects [118].

Although in situ hybridization, electrophysiology, and immunoblotting experiments confirmed the expression of NMDAR subunits mRNA and their functions in the spinal cord motor neurons [119-125], the NMDAR has not been at the center of attention in the excitotoxicity-induced motor neuron death. This is partly due to some studies showing either no or low motor neuroprotection following the application of NMDAR antagonists in ALS patients, transgenic animal models of motor neuron degeneration and in vitro set ups [126-129] or studies reporting little or no significant neuronal damage in NMDA exposure experiments [130]. On the other hand, a body of evidence suggests a direct or indirect involvement of NMDAR-dependent excitotoxicity in motor neuron degeneration in ALS. For instance, memantine, a low-affinity, noncompetitive NMDA receptor antagonist was shown to be neuroprotective against motor neuron degeneration in G93A transgenic mice [131, 132].

The cultured spinal cord motor neurons were found highly vulnerable to the NMDA induced excitotoxicity [133]. The cultured neurons isolated from the G93A mouse model of ALS were more vulnerable to NMDA excitotoxicity challenge, particularly in the presence of the Zn^{2+}ion, compared with that in wild type neuronal cultures [134]. Brunet N et al. demonstrated motor neuron degeneration in organotyptic cultures of chick embryo spinal cord treated with excitotoxins such as glutamate, NMDA, and kainate [135]. Moreover, the level of D-serine, the endogenous co-agonist of NMDARs, has been found to be elevated in the spinal cord of both sporadic and familial ALS patients and in the G93A mouse model of ALS and exacerbates motor neuron death [136]. In fact, D-serine and the activity of its degrading enzyme, the D-amino acid oxidase (compromised in classical FALS) are considered the major determinants of glutamate toxicity in ALS, suggesting an important role for NMDAR in ALS pathogenesis [137, 138]. Finally, in ALS, similar to what observed during neuronal ischemic events [139], extracellular glutamate accumulation and impaired glutamate transporter function can also exacerbate massive Ca^{2+} influx and further contribute to the AMPAR-dependent excitotoxicity induced neuronal death by depolarizing neurons and lifting the Mg^{2+} blockade of NMDARs.

Among the NMDAR subunits, GluN2B (NR2B) has been implicated in the pathogenesis of stroke, trauma, epilepsy, and neurodegenerative diseases as well as several mood disorders [71-73, 113, 114]. The c-tail of GluN2B, particularly the part localized extrasynaptically, links NMDAR to pro-death signaling pathways following inappropriate overexcitaion and massive Ca^{2+} influx (reviewed in [72, 73]). In fact, GluN2B-dependent excessive rise in intracellular Ca2+ levels triggers a variety of deleterious events leading to neuronal death. Pro-death signaling pathways and pathological mechanisms downstream of GluN2B include activation of calpain proteases and their subsequent functional outcomes (Reviewed in [140-142]), mitochondrial dysfunction and generation of reactive oxygen/nitrogen species (reviewed in [143, 144]), activation of neuronal nitric oxide synthase (nNOS) and its downstream toxic responses (reviewed in [145]), activation of stress-activated protein kinases (SAPKs) [146] , inhibition of pro-survival CREB (cAMP-response element-binding protein) transcription factor and its target genes expression, inactivation of pro-survival ERK1/2, activation of pro-death FOXOs (Reviewed in [72, 73]), and alteration in gene expression patterns such as elevation of pro-death ClCa1 gene expression [147, 148]. We have recently used a protein-DNA microarray technique to identify transcription factors binding alteration following NMDA induced excitotoxicity in cultured rat cortical neurons [60]. After screening 345 transcription factors (Tfs) against their characterized transcriptional binding sites, in NMDA treated neurons in comparison with control cells, we found two times or more increase in 21 Tfs such as ATF/CRE, ERE, FAST-1, NF-E1 (YY1), NF-E2, PAX-5, Pur-5, Stat4, ets, and SREBP1 binding sites, whereas 16 showed two times or more decrease including Smad3/4, Coup-TF, and MRE. Among those transcription factors, we studied the connection between the NMDAR dependent excitotoxicity induced activation of the lipogenic transcription factor SREBP1 and neuronal cell death. The in vitro neuronal excitotoxicity was induced by incubating cultured neurons with a transient high concentration of NMDA or oxygen glucose deprivation (OGD), a condition which simulates ischemic stroke. The excitotoxicity-induced SREBP1 activation was found NMDAR, and GluN2B dependent as AP5, a NMDAR blocker, and Ro25-6981, a specific GluN2B subunit antagonist blocked the transcription factor activation, whereas NVP-AAM077, an antagonist of the GluN2A subunit failed to do that. The excitotoxicity-induced neuronal SREBP1 activation was also Ca^{2+} and calpain dependent. We also observed SREBP1 activation in the rat MCAO model of stroke. We established a direct causative link between GluN2B dependent excitotoxicity induced SREBP1 activation and neuronal apoptosis [60]. The observed phenomenon was SREBP2 independent. In order to disrupt this deleterious causative link and provide neuroprotection, we designed a short cell penetrating bioactive peptide called "Indip". We designed the Indip peptide based on the molecular mechanism of SREBP activation.

Molecular Mechanism of SREBP1 Activation

The SREBPs are members of the basic helix–loop–helix (bHLH) leucine zipper family of transcription factors, which are best known to regulate lipid metabolism in the liver and adipose tissue. The SREBP family consists of SREBP-1a, SREBP-1c and SREBP-2 (reviewed in [149, 150]). The SREBPs are conserved from fission yeast to man. SREBP1a and 1c are produced from a single gene on chromosome 17 p11.2 from two different promoters, whereas SREBP2 is encoded from a gene on chromosome 22q13.Both SREBP1 isoforms activate transcription of genes involved in the biosynthesis of cholesterol and fatty acids, whereas SREBP2 preferentially activates target genes in cholesterol biosynthesis and metabolism pathways. The SREBPs are synthesized and located as a transmembrane protein on the ER in their premature (full length) forms and are associated with another ER membrane protein called SCAP (SREBP-cleavage-activating protein) through their C-terminal interaction. The N-terminal (sterol sensing domain) of SCAP interacts with an ER-membrane resident protein, Insig (insulin-induced gene). This interaction retains SCAP-SREBP complex in the ER. Mammalian cells contain two homologues of Insig (1 and 2) with similar functions [151]. In order to be activated as a transcription factor, the SCAP-SREBP complex (inactive) needs to be transported to the Golgi apparatus, where SREBPs are processed sequentially by two proteases, S1P (site 1 protease) and S2P (site 2 protease). The cleaved 68 KDa N-terminal of SREBPs forms active homodimers, and translocate to the nucleus in an importin-β dependent manner.After nuclear translocation they bind and regulate the expression of genes carrying sterol response element (SRE) and E-box in their promoters [149, 150, 152]. Most of these genes are involved in lipid biogenesis and metabolism as well as cellular electron transfer and respiration [153].

Insig-1 mediates feedback inhibition of cholesterol biosynthesis. When excess sterols are accumulated in the cell and the cholesterol content of membranes increases, Insig-1 sequesters the SCAP-SREBP complex in the ER or binds to3-hydroxy-3-methyl-glutaryl coenzyme A (HMG-CoA) reductase and suppresses cholesterol and lipid biosynthesis and uptake [149, 150]. A decline in the membrane cholesterol content prevents Insig-1 binding to SCAP or HMG-CoA, allowing the SREBP-SCAP complex to be transported to the Golgi apparatus for proteolytic activation and rescues the HMG-CoA from degradation, respectively. In cholesterol deprived cells, Insig-1 binds to an E3 ubiquitin ligase, gp78, (reviewed in [154]) and is targeted for polyubiquitination and subsequent degradation via the ER-associated degradation (ERAD) pathway (recently reviewed in [155, 156]). Following ubiquitination on Lys156 and Lys158, Insig-1 is degraded by the proteasome [157-159]. Two other proteins, p97 and Ubxd8 facilitate the proteasomal degradation of polyubiquitinated Insig-1 by extracting it from the ER membrane [160, 161]. Cellular stress such as hypotonic shock and ER stress also activate SREBPs via rapid turnover of Insig-1 [162]. Cholesterol treatment of cells promotes SCAP binding to Insig-1, displaces gp78 from Insig-1 and prevents its degradation resulting in inhibition of SREBP activation [159]. In the absence of cholesterol, exogenous unsaturated fatty acids prevent the degradation of ubiquitinated Insig-1 by blocking its association with the Ubxd8/p97 complex. To directly inhibit Insig-1 degradation, we designed an Insig-1–derived interference peptide (Indip) that contains the above mentioned ubiquitination sites (GEPHKFKREW) [157]. We rendered Indip membrane permeable by fusing it to the cell-membrane transduction domain of the HIV-1 Tat protein (YGRKKRRQRRR) [163]. We assumed that Indip would efficiently block Insig-1 ubiquitination and hence its degradation by the proteasome whereas a control peptide ($Indip_{K-R}$) in which the active lysine residues were switched to arginine (GEPHRFRREW) would be ineffective. As predicted, when we challenged cultured HEK cells with simvastatin to inhibit cholesterol synthesis (by activating SREBPs), Indip efficiently blocked simvastatin-induced Insig-1 ubiquitination, and degradation, as well as the subsequent SREBP1 activation, whereas the control peptide, $Indip_{K-R}$ failed to exert any effect [60]. Therefore, Indip is an effective tool to block SREBP1 activation by inhibiting Insig-1 degradation. We have also used Indip to modify lipoprotein profile in fructose-fed hamsters (Taghibiglou C et al. unpublished data).

Pathological Activation of Neuronal SREBP1: A Common Denominator in Stroke and ALS

Dysregulations of SREBPs activation in peripheral tissues-Pathological activation of SREBP1 has been previously reported in different peripheral tissues (reviewed in [152]). For instance, SREBP-1 activation has been linked to glucolipotoxic cell death in pancreatic β-cells which share common embryonic origin with neurons [164-169]. It is noteworthy that the activation of SREBP-1 has also been found in response to anaerobic and hypoxic stress in fission yeast, *Cryptococcus* neoformans [170, 171] and *Caenorhabditis elegans* [172, 173]. In fact, SREBP1 has a homologues function to an oxygen sensor [174]. Implication of SREBP-dependent lipotoxicity in the pathogenesis of obesity, and its pathological manifestations has been well established (reviewed in [175, 176]). Dysregulation of SREBPs and their downstream effectors have also been reported in prostate cancer progression [177, 178]. Overexpression of the fatty acid synthase (FAS) enzyme, a down-stream target of SREBP1 has been demonstrated in human tumors and transformed cell lines [179, 180]. Most recently, Plantier L et al. reported that overactivation of SREBPs or pulmonary lipotoxicity enhances lipogenesis in respiratory epithelial cells resulting in lung inflammation and tissue remodeling [181]. Moreover, Coxsackievirus B3 (CVB3) infection in cardiomyocyes activates the unfolded protein response and induces apoptosis through the activation of SREBP1 [182]. SREBP1 activation has been also involved in the hepatitis C virus (HCV) induced lipid accumulation and liver steatosis (reviewed in [183]). Ischemia and acute pharmacological cytotoxicity induced renal damage are associated with proximal tube lipid accumulation due to the activation of SREBPs and their downstream target genes [184-186]. Down-regulation of Insig-1 and activation of SREBP1, have also been implicated in the persistent organic pollutant (POP) exposure-induced insulin resistance syndrome in rats [187]. This is important because environmental toxins are also considered as risk factors in the pathogenesis of ALS (reviewed in [188, 189]).

Pathological activation of neuronal SREBP1- For more than four decades, the role of lipid moieties and lipid related transcription factors including SREBPs in physiology and pathophysiology of peripheral tissues has been a very attractive and productive research topic, particularly in cardiovascular and diabetes research fields. However, SREBPs have not been at the center of attention of neuroscientists and neurologists until recently, when emerging data suggested an important role for lipids in the pathogenesis of mood disorders and neurodegenerative diseases (Reviewed in [190-200]).

As discussed above, we have recently discovered a novel NMDAR-dependent signaling pathway connecting GluN2B subunit induced excitotoxicity to the activation of the lipid transcription factor SREBP1 and neuronal apoptosis in both in vitro and in vivo models of stroke [60]. This deleterious SREBP1 activation was Ca^{2+}, calpain, and time dependent, whereas it was caspase-3 independent. Excitotoxicity-induced neuronal death also up-regulated the expression of SREBP1 downstream gene targets [153] such as stearoyl-CoA desaturase (SCD) and Fatty acid synthase (FAS). It did not affect the activity of either SREBP2 or its downstream gene targets. Interestingly, incubating neurons with a high exogenous cholesterol concentration suppressed SREBP1 activation through an inhibitory feed-back response [149, 150] and resulted in neuroprotection against NMDA induced excitotoxicity (Figure 2). SREBP1 knockdown using a specific shRNA also resulted in neuroprotection against NMDA insult. More notably, Indip, a short cell penetrating bioactive peptide, demonstrated profound neuroprotection in both in vitro and in vivo excitotoxicity and stroke set ups by stabilizing Insig-1 and subsequent inhibition of SREBP1 activation (Figure 3).

More recently, we investigated the activation of the same deleterious signaling pathway in the pathogenesis of ALS using post-mortem human control and ALS spinal cord specimens as well as spinal cord samples of wild type and G93A aggressive mutant SOD1 transgenic mice [61]. Similar to stroke, we found a drastic Insig-1 degradation and SREBP1 activation in both post-mortem (FALS and SALS) and G93A spinal cord tissues. This is the first report implicating Insig-1 and SREBP1 in the pathogenesis of ALS. A significant reduction of Insig-2 has also been reported in microarray analysis of G93A mouse motor neurons [201]. Using apoptosis TUNEL assay and non-biased lactate dehydrogenase (LDH) based toxicology assay, we observed neuroprotective effects of Indip in glutamate-induced excitotoxicity in cultured G93A and wild type spinal cord neurons.

The implication of the SREBP1 transcription factor in the pathogenesis of ALS suggests that disrupting the activation of this pathway by Indip and other pharmacological and nutritional agents may provide novel therapeutic approaches to the disease.

Detailed mechanisms by which the activation of SREBP-1 leads to enhanced neuronal damage remain to be established. SREBPs are the major transcription factors that regulate the expression of a large number of genes containing SRE and E-box sequences in their promoters. The majority of these genes are involved in cellular cholesterol and lipid biogenesis and homeostasis [149, 202].

Altered lipid metabolism has recently been implicated in mediating neuronal damage in brain injury and various brain disorders [190]. Thus, it is very plausible to speculate that the activation of SREBP-1 may exert its pro-neuronal death action by altering one or more of these lipid products.

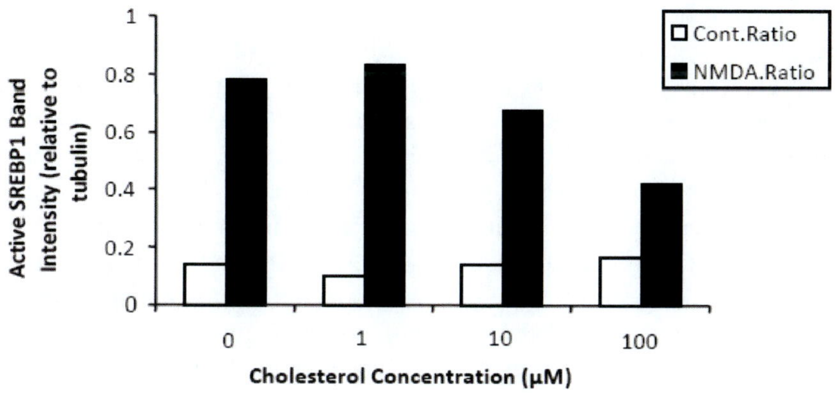

Figure 2. Cholesterol treatment suppressed NMDA-induced activation of SREBP-1 in cultured rat cortical neurons. Neurons were incubated with cholesterol at the indicated concentrations 12 h before NMDA-induced excitotoxicity. Control neurons were not exposed to NMDA. Cell lysates were collected 6 h post excitotoxicity and subjected to immunoblotting for SREBP1 and tubulin.

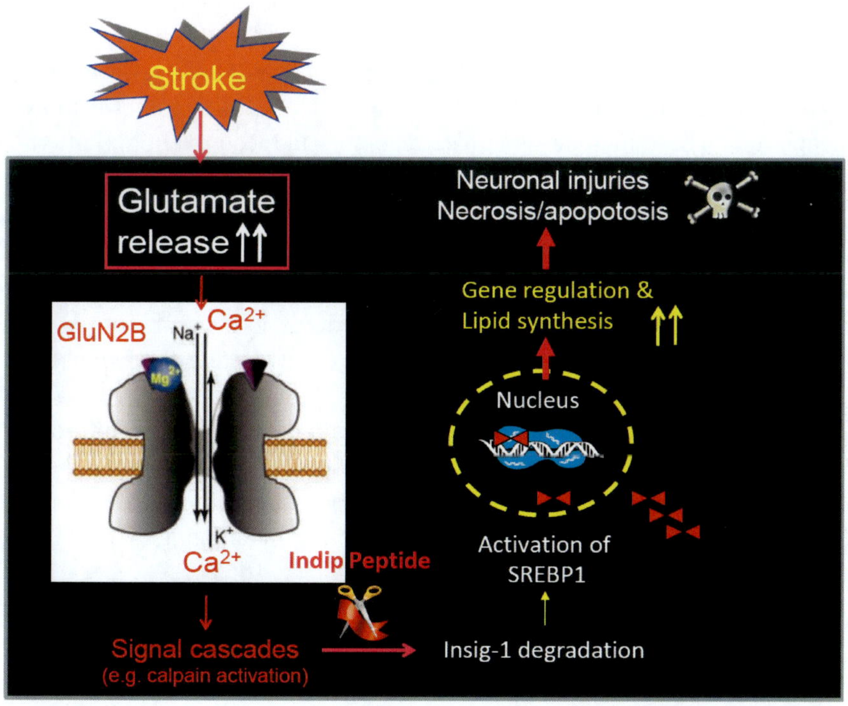

Figure 3. GluN2B dependent excitotoxicity-induced neuronal death in stroke- Massive glutamate release and inefficient take up by glia cells cause an excessive Ca2+ influx and activation of calcium-dependent deleterious pathways such as calpain proteases. It also mediates Insig-1 degradation resulting in the activation of SREBP1 and neuronal apoptosis. Indip peptide by stabilizing Insig-1 prevents SREBP1 activation and exerts neuroprotection in both in vitro and in vivo models of stroke.

In fact, using radiolabeled lipid precursors, we have observed neuronal lipid profile alterations following NMDA-induced excitotoxicity (Taghibiglou C. unpublished data).

Moreover, SREBP-1 regulates the expression of a number of SRE and E-box–containing genes which may not be directly involved in lipid metabolism, including G proteins [203], voltage-gated ion channels [204] and other newly identified potential target genes [205]. Thus, SREBP-1 may also contribute to neuronal damage via a mechanism independent of alterations in lipid metabolism. SREBP1 is also activated in an Akt-dependent manner via mTORC1 pathway to mediate cell growth [206, 207]. However, whether inactivation of SREBP-1 incirectly contributes to its neuroprotective effects by attenuating cell growth and allowing better management of vital cellular resources remains to be determined.

Although the question of how the activation of SREBP1 leads to neuronal apoptosis still remains to be answered, there is no doubt that neuronal inhibition or suppression of this lipid transcription factor exerts neuroprotection. This fact opens up numerous opportunities for using therapeutic and nutritional agents to disrupt pathways upstream or downstream of SREBP1 in order to improve survival and quality of life in ALS patients.

In the last section of this review, we will attempt to link novel emerging research results with our findings on excitotoxcity induced SREBP1 activation and neuronal death in ALS.

Putting the Pieces of Puzzle Together

The precise pathogenesis of ALS still remains unclear. However, emerging evidence obtained from studies using animal models has proposed several hypotheses to explain motor neuron degeneration. These include glutamate receptors-induced excitotoxicity, hypoxia [82] and oxidative stress [208]. Recently hypoxia and hypoxia-responsive genes, vascular alteration, and spinal hypoperfusion have been implicated in the pathogenesis of ALS [209-212]. Furthermore, in short oxygen deprivation challenges, motor neurons have been proven to be more vulnerable compared to other spinal and central neurons [213, 214].

These findings suggest that chronic hypoxia is involved in the pathology of ALS. We and the others have demonstrated that hypoxia and anoxia activate the lipid transcription factor, SREBP1, or its homologues in a variety of cell and animal models [170, 171, 173]. More importantly, we provided evidence that transient oxygen deprivation in cultured neurons and the rat brain induces neuronal excitotoxicity via the GluN2B subunit of NMDARs leading to the activation of SREBP1 and neuronal death. We demonstrated drastic neuroprotection by disrupting the activation of SREBP1 using indip peptide (stabilizing Insig-1) or exogenous cholesterol (feed-back inhibition) [60].

Activation of the same pathway has been reported in ALS further confirming the important roles of hypoxia and excitotoxicity in the pathogenesis of ALS. Neuroprotective effects of the Insig-1 derived interference peptide (Indip) against glutamate-induced excitotoxicity in cultured spinal cord neurons suggest possibilities for lipid and SREBP1-related therapeutic interventions in ALS.

This notion is supported by several pieces of evidence: It has been shown that excitotoxicity alters cholesterol biosynthetic and transport pathways in the rat hippocampus after kinate excitotoxicity [215, 216]. In line with this finding, Sodero and colleagues have recently demonstrated that glutamate-mediated excitotoxicity induces a small but significant cholesterol loss from the membrane of hippocampal neurons. The conversion of insoluble membrane (synaptic) cholesterol to the soluble metabolite 24S-hydroxycholesterol [217] and its release to the extra cellular area is NMDAR and Ca^{2+} dependent [218]. Appropriate and physiological regulation of cellular cholesterol homeostasis particularly in the plasma membrane is vital for all cell types including neurons [219].

Following excitotoxicity, the depleted cholesterol should be replaced by neighboring astrocytes. Any failure or inefficiency of glial cells in supplying lipid or scarcity of exogenous cholesterol resources may trigger the activation of neuronal SREBPs which is proven to be deleterious [60]. It is noteworthy that neurodegenerative disorders including ALS are age-dependent diseases and cholesterol synthesis rate in the human brain (hippocampus) declines with aging [220]. These findings go well with recent reports on beneficial effects of high fat diet in animal models of ALS [221] as well as ALS patients [62, 222].

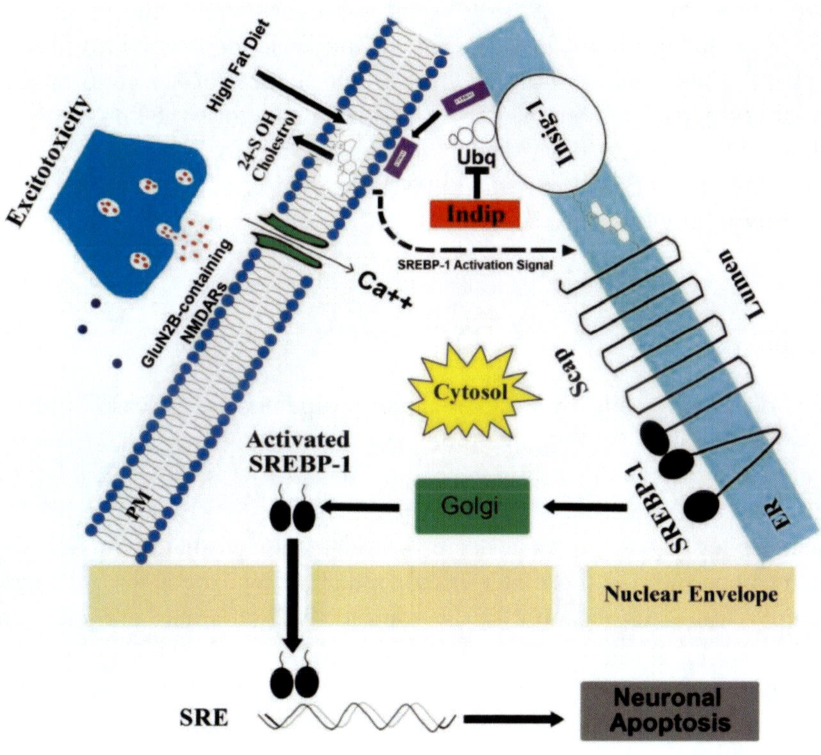

Figure 4. Hypothetical mechanism for the SREBP1 activation induced motor neuron apoptosis in ALS-Excessive glutamate in the synaptic cleft mediates massive $Ca2^+$ influx through the GluN2B-containing NMDA receptors. Following the excitotoxic insult, about 10% of insoluble cholesterol content of the plasma membrane is converted to soluble 24-S-OH cholesterol and diffused out of the membrane. The decreased plasma membrane cholesterol content triggers demand for cholesterol synthesis by the Insig-1 poly ubiquitination and degradation. Then SCAP –SREBP1 complex is transported to the Golgi apparatus, where the N-terminal of SREBP1 (active form) cleaved and then transported to the nucleus to regulate SRE and E-box containing genes causing apoptosis. Indip and high fat diet by disrupting this pathway exert neuroprotection.

In fact, growing evidence suggest that dyslipidemia (hypercholesterolemia/ hypertriglyceridemia) may be a protective factor in ALS patients [222-224], whereas the exacerbation of symptoms has been linked to lower serum lipids [225].

It has recently been reported that the G93A mouse model of ALS shows hypolipidemia at the peri-symptomatic stage [226] and caloric restriction shortens its life span [227]. Moreover, lipoic acid supplement therapy and hyperlipidemia which suppress SREBP1 activation [228] have shown beneficial effects in ALS animal model and patients, respectively [222, 229]. Treatment with statins which activates SREBPs worsened the outcome [230]. It is noteworthy that ALS-like symptoms have also been reported in some patients taking cholesterol lowering drugs [231].

Consistent to the beneficial effects of high fat diet and dyslipidemia in ALS which may attenuate hypoxia and excitotoxicity-induced SREBP1 activation in motor neurons through a feed-back inhibition mechanism, the short peptide Indip protects spinal cord neurons (in an in vitro model of ALS) by stabilizing Insig-1 and subsequent inhibition of the transcription factor [61]. In vivo studies are required to evaluate and examine the effectiveness of Indip in animal models of motor neuron diseases. Overall our studies further confirm that SREBP1 activation is an essential step in the NMDAR-mediated motor neuron death. They also indicate that any therapeutic or dietary interventions in pathways leading to the inhibition or attenuation of neuronal SREBP1 activation may have a therapeutic/neuroprotective potential in ALS treatment (Figure 4).

Conclusion

ALS is a devastating and multifactorial neurodegenerative disease, surrounded with countless unknowns, with no cure at this time, despite enormous research. Excitotoxicity and hypoxia are among factors implicated in the pathogenesis of ALS. We have demonstrated that both of these factors activate the lipid transcription factor, SREBP1, in a NMDA receptor dependent manner leading to neuronal death. We also showed that disrupting the SREBP1 activation pathway by Indip, a short interfering peptide, or by exogenous lipid administration (via an inhibitory feed-back response) is neuroprotective. This may provide a mechanistic explanation for recent reports on the beneficial effects of high fat diet for ALS patients. Finally, we suggest that attenuating SREBP1 activation may have a therapeutic value in ALS. Further investigations including in vivo studies are required to test the effectiveness of Indip in experimental motor neuron diseases as well as other models of neurodegeneration.

References

[1] Rowland, L.P. and Shneider, N.A. Amyotrophic lateral sclerosis. *N Engl J. Med.* 344, 1688-1700 (2001).

[2] Logroscino, G., *et al.* Incidence of amyotrophic lateral sclerosis in Europe. *J. Neurol. Neurosurg. Psychiatry* 81, 385-390 (2010).

[3] Byrne, S., *et al.* Rate of familial amyotrophic laterals sclerosis: a systematic review and meta-analysis. *J. Neurol. Neurosurg. Psychiatry* 82, 623-627 (2011).

[4] Hardiman, O., van den Berg, L.H. and Kiernan, M.C. Clinical diagnosis and management of amyotrophic lateral sclerosis. *Nat. Rev. Neurol.* 7, 639-649 (2011).

[5] Kiernan, M.C., *et al.* Amyotrophic lateral sclerosis. *Lancet* 377, 942-955 (2011).

[6] Andersen, P.M. and Al-Chalabi, A. Clinical genetics of amyotrophic lateral sclerosis: what do we really know? *Nat. Rev. Neurol.* 7, 603-615 (2011).

[7] Dion, P.A., Daoud, H. and Rouleau, G.A. Genetics of motor neuron disorders: new insights into pathogenic mechanisms. *Nat. Rev. Genet.* 10, 769-782 (2009).

[8] Rosen, D.R., *et al.* Mutations in Cu/Zn superoxide dismutase gene are associated with familial amyotrophic lateral sclerosis. *Nature* 362, 59-62 (1993).

[9] Kawamata, H. and Manfredi, G. Import, maturation, and function of SOD1 and its copper chaperone CCS in the mitochondrial intermembrane space. *Antioxid. Redox. Signal.* 13, 1375-1384 (2010).

[10] Barber, S.C. and Shaw, P.J. Oxidative stress in ALS: key role in motor neuron injury and therapeutic target. *Free Radic. Biol. Med.* 48, 629-641 (2010).

[11] Da Cruz, S. and Cleveland, D.W. Understanding the role of TDP-43 and FUS/TLS in ALS and beyond. *Curr Opin Neurobiol*21, 904-919 (2011).

[12] Gitler, A.D. and Shorter, J. RNA-binding proteins with prion-like domains in ALS and FTLD-U. *Prion.* 5, 179-187 (2011).

[13] Mackenzie, I.R., Rademakers, R. and Neumann, M. TDP-43 and FUS in amyotrophic lateral sclerosis and frontotemporal dementia. *Lancet Neurol.* 9, 995-1007 (2010).

[14] Udan, M. and Baloh, R.H. Implications of the prion-related Q/N domains in TDP-43 and FUS. *Prion.* 5, 1-5 (2011).

[15] Kwiatkowski, T.J., Jr., *et al.* Mutations in the FUS/TLS gene on chromosome 16 cause familial amyotrophic lateral sclerosis. *Science* 323, 1205-1208 (2009).

[16] Vance, C., *et al.* Mutations in FUS, an RNA processing protein, cause familial amyotrophic lateral sclerosis type 6. *Science*323, 1208-1211 (2009).

[17] Couthouis, J., *et al.* A yeast functional screen predicts new candidate ALS disease genes. *Proc. Natl. Acad. Sci. U S A*108, 20881-20890 (2011).

[18] Deng, H.X., *et al.* Mutations in UBQLN2 cause dominant X-linked juvenile and adult-onset ALS and ALS/dementia. *Nature* 477, 211-215 (2011).

[19] Nishimura, A.L., Al-Chalabi, A. and Zatz, M. A common founder for amyotrophic lateral sclerosis type 8 (ALS8) in the Brazilian population. *Hum. Genet.* 118, 499-500 (2005).

[20] Nishimura, A.L., *et al.* A mutation in the vesicle-trafficking protein VAPB causes late-onset spinal muscular atrophy and amyotrophic lateral sclerosis. *Am. J. Hum. Genet.* 75, 822-831 (2004).

[21] Greenway, M.J., *et al.* ANG mutations segregate with familial and 'sporadic' amyotrophic lateral sclerosis. *Nat. Genet.* 38, 411-413 (2006).

[22] Maruyama, H., *et al.* Mutations of optineurin in amyotrophic lateral sclerosis. *Nature* 465, 223-226 (2010).

[23] Boillee, S., Vande Velde, C. and Cleveland, D.W. ALS: a disease of motor neurons and their nonneuronal neighbors. *Neuron*5 2, 39-59 (2006).

[24] Pasinelli, P. and Brown, R.H. Molecular biology of amyotrophic lateral sclerosis: insights from genetics. *Nat. Rev. Neurosci.* 7, 710-723 (2006).

[25] Strong, M.J., Kesavapany, S. and Pant, H.C. The pathobiology of amyotrophic lateral sclerosis: a proteinopathy? *J. Neuropathol. Exp. Neurol.* 64, 649-664 (2005).

[26] Chio, A., Benzi, G., Dossena, M., Mutani, R. and Mora, G. Severely increased risk of amyotrophic lateral sclerosis among Italian professional football players. *Brain* 128, 472-476 (2005).

[27] Harwood, C.A., McDermott, C.J. and Shaw, P.J. Physical activity as an exogenous risk factor in motor neuron disease (MND): a review of the evidence. *Amyotroph. Lateral Scler.*10, 191-204 (2009).

[28] Wicks, P., *et al.* Three soccer playing friends with simultaneous amyotrophic lateral sclerosis. *Amyotroph. Lateral Scler.* 8, 177-179 (2007).

[29] Kasarskis, E.J., *et al.* Clinical aspects of ALS in Gulf War veterans. *Amyotroph. Lateral Scler.* 10, 35-41 (2009).

[30] Weisskopf, M.G., *et al.* Prospective study of military service and mortality from ALS. *Neurology* 64, 32-37 (2005).

[31] Alonso, A., Logroscino, G. and Hernan, M.A. Smoking and the risk of amyotrophic lateral sclerosis: a systematic review and meta-analysis. *J. Neurol. Neurosurg. Psychiatry* 81, 1249-1252 (2010).

[32] Gallo, V., *et al.* Smoking and risk for amyotrophic lateral sclerosis: analysis of the EPIC cohort. *Ann. Neurol.* 65, 378-385 (2009).

[33] Wang, H., *et al.* Smoking and risk of amyotrophic lateral sclerosis: a pooled analysis of 5 prospective cohorts. *Arch. Neurol.* 68, 207-213 (2011).

[34] Caller, T.A., *et al.* Spatial clustering of amyotrophic lateral sclerosis and the potential role of BMAA. *Amyotroph. Lateral Scler.* 13, 25-32 (2012).

[35] Chiu, A.S., Gehringer, M.M., Welch, J.H. and Neilan, B.A. Does alpha-amino-beta-methylaminopropionic acid (BMAA) play a role in neurodegeneration? *Int. J. Environ. Res. Public. Health* 8, 3728-3746 (2011).

[36] Contrusciere, V., Paradisi, S., Matteucci, A. and Malchiodi-Albedi, F. Branched-chain amino acids induce neurotoxicity in rat cortical cultures. *Neurotox. Res.* 17, 392-398 (2010).

[37] Cox, P.A. and Sacks, O.W. Cycad neurotoxins, consumption of flying foxes, and ALS-PDC disease in Guam. *Neurology*58, 956-959 (2002).

[38] Cozzolino, M. and Carri, M.T. Mitochondrial dysfunction in ALS. *Prog. Neurobiol.* 97, 54-66 (2012).

[39] Duffy, L.M., Chapman, A.L., Shaw, P.J. and Grierson, A.J. Review: The role of mitochondria in the pathogenesis of amyotrophic lateral sclerosis. *Neuropathol. Appl. Neurobiol.* 37, 336-352 (2011).

[40] Martin, L.J. Mitochondrial pathobiology in ALS. *J. Bioenerg. Biomembr.* 43, 569-579 (2011).

[41] Okamoto, K., Fujita, Y. and Mizuno, Y. Pathology of protein synthesis and degradation systems in ALS. *Neuropathology* 30, 189-193 (2010).

[42] Kanekura, K., Suzuki, H., Aiso, S. and Matsuoka, M. ER stress and unfolded protein response in amyotrophic lateral sclerosis. *Mol. Neurobiol.* 39, 81-89 (2009).

[43] De Vos, K.J., Grierson, A.J., Ackerley, S. and Miller, C.C. Role of axonal transport in neurodegenerative diseases. *Annu. Rev. Neurosci.* 31, 151-173 (2008).

[44] Philips, T. and Robberecht, W. Neuroinflammation in amyotrophic lateral sclerosis: role of glial activation in motor neuron disease. *Lancet Neurol.* 10, 253-263 (2011).

[45] Van Den Bosch, L. and Robberecht, W. Crosstalk between astrocytes and motor neurons: what is the message? *Exp. Neurol.* 211, 1-6 (2008).

[46] Grosskreutz, J., Van Den Bosch, L. and Keller, B.U. Calcium dysregulation in amyotrophic lateral sclerosis. *Cell Calcium* 47, 165-174 (2010).

[47] Zhong, Z., *et al.* Activated protein C therapy slows ALS-like disease in mice by transcriptionally inhibiting SOD1 in motor neurons and microglia cells. *J. Clin. Invest.* 119, 3437-3449 (2009).

[48] Vargas, M.R., Johnson, D.A., Sirkis, D.W., Messing, A. and Johnson, J.A. Nrf2 activation in astrocytes protects against neurodegeneration in mouse models of familial amyotrophic lateral sclerosis. *J. Neurosci.* 28, 13574-13581 (2008).

[49] Kiaei, M. Peroxisome Proliferator-Activated Receptor-gamma in Amyotrophic Lateral Sclerosis and Huntington's Disease. *PPAR Res.* 2008, 418765 (2008).

[50] Eve, D.J., Dennis, J.S. and Citron, B.A. Transcription factor p53 in degenerating spinal cords. *Brain Res.* 1150, 174-181 (2007).

[51] Vlug, A.S., *et al.* ATF3 expression precedes death of spinal motoneurons in amyotrophic lateral sclerosis-SOD1 transgenic mice and correlates with c-Jun phosphorylation, CHOP expression, somato-dendritic ubiquitination and Golgi fragmentation. *Eur. J. Neurosci.* 22, 1881-1894 (2005).

[52] Jaarsma, D., *et al.* Induction of c-Jun immunoreactivity in spinal cord and brainstem neurons in a transgenic mouse model for amyotrophic lateral sclerosis. *Neurosci. Lett.* 219, 179-182 (1996).

[53] Zhai, J., Lin, H., Canete-Soler, R. and Schlaepfer, W.W. HoxB2 binds mutant SOD1 and is altered in transgenic model of ALS. *Hum. Mol. Genet.* 14, 2629-2640 (2005).

[54] Batulan, Z., *et al.* High threshold for induction of the stress response in motor neurons is associated with failure to activate HSF1. *J. Neurosci.* 23, 5789-5798 (2003).

[55] Chung, Y.H., Joo, K.M., Lee, Y.J., Kim, M.J. and Cha, C.I. Reactive astrocytes express cAMP-response-element-binding protein (CREB) binding protein (CBP) in the central nervous system of transgenic mice expressing a human Cu/Zn superoxide dismutase mutation. *Neurosci. Lett.* 343, 159-162 (2003).

[56] Migheli, A., Piva, R., Atzori, C., Troost, D. and Schiffer, D. c-Jun, JNK/SAPK kinases and transcription factor NF-kappa B are selectively activated in astrocytes, but not motor neurons, in amyotrophic lateral sclerosis. *J. Neuropathol. Exp. Neurol.* 56, 1314-1322 (1997).

[57] Swarup, V., *et al.* Deregulation of TDP-43 in amyotrophic lateral sclerosis triggers nuclear factor kappaB-mediated pathogenic pathways. *J. Exp. Med.* 208, 2429-2447 (2011).

[58] Valente, T., Mancera, P., Tusell, J.M., Serratosa, J. and Saura, J. C/EBPbeta expression in activated microglia in amyotrophic lateral sclerosis. *Neurobiol. Aging.* (2011).

[59] Zhang, Z., Yan, J., Chang, Y., ShiDu Yan, S. and Shi, H. Hypoxia inducible factor-1 as a target for neurodegenerative diseases. *Curr. Med. Chem.* 18, 4335-4343 (2011).

[60] Taghibiglou, C., *et al.* Role of NMDA receptor-dependent activation of SREBP1 in excitotoxic and ischemic neuronal injuries. *Nat. Med.* 15, 1399-1406 (2009).

[61] Taghibiglou, C., Lu, J., Mackenzie, I.R., Wang, Y.T. and Cashman, N.R. Sterol regulatory element binding protein-1 (SREBP1) activation in motor neurons in excitotoxicity and amyotrophic lateral sclerosis (ALS): Indip, a potential therapeutic peptide. *Biochem. Biophys. Res. Commun.* 413, 159-163 (2011).

[62] Dupuis, L., Pradat, P.F., Ludolph, A.C. and Loeffler, J.P. Energy metabolism in amyotrophic lateral sclerosis. *Lancet Neurol.* 10, 75-82 (2011).

[63] Kim, K., *et al.* Role of excitatory amino acid transporter-2 (EAAT2) and glutamate in neurodegeneration: opportunities for developing novel therapeutics. *J. Cell Physiol.* 226, 2484-2493 (2011).
[64] Maragakis, N.J., *et al.* Glutamate transporter expression and function in human glial progenitors. *Glia* 45, 133-143 (2004).
[65] Meldrum, B. and Garthwaite, J. Excitatory amino acid neurotoxicity and neurodegenerative disease. *Trends Pharmacol. Sci.* 11, 379-387 (1990).
[66] Van Den Bosch, L., Van Damme, P., Bogaert, E. and Robberecht, W. The role of excitotoxicity in the pathogenesis of amyotrophic lateral sclerosis. *Biochim. Biophys. Acta* 1762, 1068-1082 (2006).
[67] Curtis, D.R., Phillis, J.W. and Watkins, J.C. Chemical excitation of spinal neurones. *Nature* 183, 611-612 (1959).
[68] Lucas, D.R. and Newhouse, J.P. The toxic effect of sodium L-glutamate on the inner layers of the retina. *AMA Arch. Ophthalmol.* 58, 193-201 (1957).
[69] Choi, D.W. Ionic dependence of glutamate neurotoxicity. *J. Neurosci.* 7, 369-379 (1987).
[70] Benarroch, E.E. NMDA receptors: recent insights and clinical correlations. *Neurology* 76, 1750-1757 (2011).
[71] Gladding, C.M. and Raymond, L.A. Mechanisms underlying NMDA receptor synaptic/extrasynaptic distribution and function. *Mol. Cell Neurosci.* 48, 308-320 (2011).
[72] Hardingham, G.E. Coupling of the NMDA receptor to neuroprotective and neurodestructive events. *Biochem. Soc. Trans.* 37, 1147-1160 (2009).
[73] Hardingham, G.E. and Bading, H. Synaptic versus extrasynaptic NMDA receptor signalling: implications for neurodegenerative disorders. *Nat. Rev. Neurosci.* 11, 682-696 (2010).
[74] Lai, T.W., Shyu, W.C. and Wang, Y.T. Stroke intervention pathways: NMDA receptors and beyond. *Trends Mol. Med.* 17, 266-275 (2011).
[75] Quinlan, K.A. Links between electrophysiological and molecular pathology of amyotrophic lateral sclerosis. *Integr. Comp. Biol.* 51, 913-925 (2011).
[76] Rothstein, J.D., *et al.* Abnormal excitatory amino acid metabolism in amyotrophic lateral sclerosis. *Ann. Neurol.* 28, 18-25 (1990).
[77] Shaw, P.J., Forrest, V., Ince, P.G., Richardson, J.P. and Wastell, H.J. CSF and plasma amino acid levels in motor neuron disease: elevation of CSF glutamate in a subset of patients. *Neurodegeneration* 4, 209-216 (1995).
[78] Spreux-Varoquaux, O., *et al.* Glutamate levels in cerebrospinal fluid in amyotrophic lateral sclerosis: a reappraisal using a new HPLC method with coulometric detection in a large cohort of patients. *J. Neurol. Sci.* 193, 73-78 (2002).
[79] Tarasiuk, J., Kulakowska, A., Drozdowski, W., Kornhuber, J. and Lewczuk, P. CSF markers in amyotrophic lateral sclerosis. *J. Neural. Transm.*
[80] Yanez, M., *et al.* CSF from amyotrophic lateral sclerosis patients produces glutamate independent death of rat motor brain cortical neurons: protection by resveratrol but not riluzole. *Brain Res.* 1423, 77-86 (2011).
[81] Rothstein, J.D., Martin, L.J. and Kuncl, R.W. Decreased glutamate transport by the brain and spinal cord in amyotrophic lateral sclerosis. *N Engl. J. Med.* 326, 1464-1468 (1992).

[82] Rothstein, J.D., Van Kammen, M., Levey, A.I., Martin, L.J. and Kuncl, R.W. Selective loss of glial glutamate transporter GLT-1 in amyotrophic lateral sclerosis. *Ann. Neurol.* 38, 73-84 (1995).

[83] Vanoni, C., *et al.* Increased internalisation and degradation of GLT-1 glial glutamate transporter in a cell model for familial amyotrophic lateral sclerosis (ALS). *J. Cell Sci.* 117, 5417-5426 (2004).

[84] Wilson, J.M., Khabazian, I., Pow, D.V., Craig, U.K. and Shaw, C.A. Decrease in glial glutamate transporter variants and excitatory amino acid receptor down-regulation in a murine model of ALS-PDC. *Neuromolecular Med.* 3, 105-118 (2003).

[85] Yin, H.Z., Tang, D.T. and Weiss, J.H. Intrathecal infusion of a Ca(2+)-permeable AMPA channel blocker slows loss of both motor neurons and of the astrocyte glutamate transporter, GLT-1 in a mutant SOD1 rat model of ALS. *Exp. Neurol.* 207, 177-185 (2007).

[86] Ilieva, H.S., *et al.* Mutant dynein (Loa) triggers proprioceptive axon loss that extends survival only in the SOD1 ALS model with highest motor neuron death. *Proc. Natl. Acad. Sci. U S A*105, 12599-12604 (2008).

[87] Sun, H., Kawahara, Y., Ito, K., Kanazawa, I. and Kwak, S. Slow and selective death of spinal motor neurons in vivo by intrathecal infusion of kainic acid: implications for AMPA receptor-mediated excitotoxicity in ALS. *J. Neurochem.* 98, 782-791 (2006).

[88] Couratier, P., Hugon, J., Sindou, P., Vallat, J.M. and Dumas, M. Cell culture evidence for neuronal degeneration in amyotrophic lateral sclerosis being linked to glutamate AMPA/kainate receptors. *Lancet* 341, 265-268 (1993).

[89] Tikka, T.M., *et al.* Minocycline prevents neurotoxicity induced by cerebrospinal fluid from patients with motor neurone disease. *Brain* 125, 722-731 (2002).

[90] Corona, J.C. and Tapia, R. AMPA receptor activation, but not the accumulation of endogenous extracellular glutamate, induces paralysis and motor neuron death in rat spinal cord in vivo. *J. Neurochem.* 89, 988-997 (2004).

[91] Corona, J.C., Tovar-y-Romo, L.B. and Tapia, R. Glutamate excitotoxicity and therapeutic targets for amyotrophic lateral sclerosis. *Expert Opin. The.r Targets* 11, 1415-1428 (2007).

[92] Anggono, V. and Huganir, R.L. Regulation of AMPA receptor trafficking and synaptic plasticity. *Curr. Opin. Neurobiol.*

[93] Wright, A. and Vissel, B. The essential role of AMPA receptor GluR2 subunit RNA editing in the normal and diseased brain. *Front Mol. Neurosci.* 5, 34 (2012).

[94] Peng, P.L., *et al.* ADAR2-dependent RNA editing of AMPA receptor subunit GluR2 determines vulnerability of neurons in forebrain ischemia. *Neuron* 49, 719-733 (2006).

[95] Brusa, R., *et al.* Early-onset epilepsy and postnatal lethality associated with an editing-deficient GluR-B allele in mice. *Science* 270, 1677-1680 (1995).

[96] Higuchi, M., *et al.* Point mutation in an AMPA receptor gene rescues lethality in mice deficient in the RNA-editing enzyme ADAR2. *Nature* 406, 78-81 (2000).

[97] Cenci, C., *et al.* Down-regulation of RNA editing in pediatric astrocytomas: ADAR2 editing activity inhibits cell migration and proliferation. *J. Biol. Chem.* 283, 7251-7260 (2008).

[98] Maas, S., Patt, S., Schrey, M. and Rich, A. Underediting of glutamate receptor GluR-B mRNA in malignant gliomas. *Proc. Natl. Acad. Sci. U S A*98, 14687-14692 (2001).

[99] Kawahara, Y., *et al.* Glutamate receptors: RNA editing and death of motor neurons. *Nature* 427, 801 (2004).

[100] Kwak, S. and Kawahara, Y. Deficient RNA editing of GluR2 and neuronal death in amyotropic lateral sclerosis. *J. Mol. Med. (Berl)*83, 110-120 (2005).

[101] Tortarolo, M., *et al.* Glutamate AMPA receptors change in motor neurons of SOD1G93A transgenic mice and their inhibition by a noncompetitive antagonist ameliorates the progression of amytrophic lateral sclerosis-like disease. *J. Neurosci. Res.* 83, 134-146 (2006).

[102] Corona, J.C. and Tapia, R. Ca2+-permeable AMPA receptors and intracellular Ca2+ determine motoneuron vulnerability in rat spinal cord in vivo. *Neuropharmacology* 52, 1219-1228 (2007).

[103] Sasabe, J. and Aiso, S. Aberrant control of motoneuronal excitability in amyotrophic lateral sclerosis: excitatory glutamate/D-serine vs. inhibitory glycine/gamma-aminobutanoic acid (GABA). *Chem. Biodivers.* 7, 1479-1490 (2010).

[104] Bliss, T. and Schoepfer, R. Neuroscience. Controlling the ups and downs of synaptic strength. *Science* 304, 973-974 (2004).

[105] Paoletti, P. Molecular basis of NMDA receptor functional diversity. *Eur J. Neurosci.* 33, 1351-1365 (2011).

[106] Seeburg, P.H., *et al.* The NMDA receptor channel: molecular design of a coincidence detector. *Recent Prog. Horm. Res.* 50, 19-34 (1995).

[107] Panatier, A., *et al.* Glia-derived D-serine controls NMDA receptor activity and synaptic memory. *Cell* 125, 775-784 (2006).

[108] Bliss, T.V. and Collingridge, G.L. A synaptic model of memory: long-term potentiation in the hippocampus. *Nature* 361, 31-39 (1993).

[109] Collingridge, G.L., Isaac, J.T. and Wang, Y.T. Receptor trafficking and synaptic plasticity. *Nat. Rev. Neurosci.* 5, 952-962 (2004).

[110] Thomas, G.M. and Huganir, R.L. MAPK cascade signalling and synaptic plasticity. *Nat. Rev. Neurosci.* 5, 173-183 (2004).

[111] Arundine, M. and Tymianski, M. Molecular mechanisms of glutamate-dependent neurodegeneration in ischemia and traumatic brain injury. *Cell Mol. Life Sci.* 61, 657-668 (2004).

[112] Kalia, L.V., Kalia, S.K. and Salter, M.W. NMDA receptors in clinical neurology: excitatory times ahead. *Lancet Neurol.* 7, 742-755 (2008).

[113] Lipton, S.A. Paradigm shift in neuroprotection by NMDA receptor blockade: memantine and beyond. *Nat. Rev. Drug Discov.* 5, 160-170 (2006).

[114] Milnerwood, A.J. and Raymond, L.A. Early synaptic pathophysiology in neurodegeneration: insights from Huntington's disease. *Trends Neurosci.* 33, 513-523 (2010).

[115] Hardingham, G.E., Fukunaga, Y. and Bading, H. Extrasynaptic NMDARs oppose synaptic NMDARs by triggering CREB shut-off and cell death pathways. *Nat. Neurosci.* 5, 405-414 (2002).

[116] Yano, S., Tokumitsu, H. and Soderling, T.R. Calcium promotes cell survival through CaM-K kinase activation of the protein-kinase-B pathway. *Nature* 396, 584-587 (1998).

[117] Paoletti, P. and Neyton, J. NMDA receptor subunits: function and pharmacology. *Curr. Opin. Pharmacol.* 7, 39-47 (2007).

[118] Samarasinghe, S., Virgo, L. and de Belleroche, J. Distribution of the N-methyl-D-aspartate glutamate receptor subunit NR2A in control and amyotrophic lateral sclerosis spinal cord. *Brain Res.* 727, 233-237 (1996).

[119] Abdrachmanova, G., Teisinger, J., Vlachova, V. and Vyklicky, L., Jr. Molecular and functional properties of synaptically activated NMDA receptors in neonatal motoneurons in rat spinal cord slices. *Eur. J. Neurosci.* 12, 955-963 (2000).

[120] Hori, Y. and Kanda, K. Developmental alterations in NMDA receptor-mediated currents in neonatal rat spinal motoneurons. *Neurosci. Lett.* 205, 99-102 (1996).

[121] MacLean, J.N., Schmidt, B.J. and Hochman, S. NMDA receptor activation triggers voltage oscillations, plateau potentials and bursting in neonatal rat lumbar motoneurons in vitro. *Eur. J. Neurosci.* 9, 2702-2711 (1997).

[122] Petralia, R.S., Yokotani, N. and Wenthold, R.J. Light and electron microscope distribution of the NMDA receptor subunit NMDAR1 in the rat nervous system using a selective anti-peptide antibody. *J. Neurosci.* 14, 667-696 (1994).

[123] Shibata, T., Watanabe, M., Ichikawa, R., Inoue, Y. and Koyanagi, T. Different expressions of alpha-amino-3-hydroxy-5-methyl-4-isoxazole propionic acid and N-methyl-D-aspartate receptor subunit mRNAs between visceromotor and somatomotor neurons of the rat lumbosacral spinal cord. *J. Comp. Neurol.* 404, 172-182 (1999).

[124] Tolle, T.R., Berthele, A., Laurie, D.J., Seeburg, P.H. and Zieglgansberger, W. Cellular and subcellular distribution of NMDAR1 splice variant mRNA in the rat lumbar spinal cord. *Eur. J. Neurosci.* 7, 1235-1244 (1995).

[125] Tolle, T.R., Berthele, A., Zieglgansberger, W., Seeburg, P.H. and Wisden, W. The differential expression of 16 NMDA and non-NMDA receptor subunits in the rat spinal cord and in periaqueductal gray. *J. Neurosci.* 13, 5009-5028 (1993).

[126] Blin, O., *et al.* A controlled one-year trial of dextromethorphan in amyotrophic lateral sclerosis. *Clin Neuropharmacol*19, 189-192 (1996).

[127] Boyce, S., *et al.* Onset and progression of motor deficits in motor neuron degeneration (mnd) mice are unaltered by the glycine/NMDA receptor antagonist L-701,324 or the MAO-B inhibitor R(-)-deprenyl. *Exp. Neurol.* 155, 49-58 (1999).

[128] Gredal, O., *et al.* A clinical trial of dextromethorphan in amyotrophic lateral sclerosis. *Acta Neurol. Scand.* 96, 8-13 (1997).

[129] Krieger, C., Perry, T.L., Hansen, S., Mitsumoto, H. and Honore, T. Excitatory amino acid receptor antagonist in murine motoneuron disease (the wobbler mouse). *Can. J. Neurol. Sci.* 19, 462-465 (1992).

[130] King, A.E., *et al.* Excitotoxicity mediated by non-NMDA receptors causes distal axonopathy in long-term cultured spinal motor neurons. *Eur. J. Neurosci.* 26, 2151-2159 (2007).

[131] Joo, I.S., Hwang, D.H., Seok, J.I., Shin, S.K. and Kim, S.U. Oral administration of memantine prolongs survival in a transgenic mouse model of amyotrophic lateral sclerosis. *J. Clin. Neurol.* 3, 181-186 (2007).

[132] Wang, R. and Zhang, D. Memantine prolongs survival in an amyotrophic lateral sclerosis mouse model. *Eur. J. Neurosci.* 22, 2376-2380 (2005).

[133] Urushitani, M., *et al.* N-methyl-D-aspartate receptor-mediated mitochondrial Ca(2+) overload in acute excitotoxic motor neuron death: a mechanism distinct from chronic neurotoxicity after Ca(2+) influx. *J. Neurosci. Res.* 63, 377-387 (2001).

[134] Nutini, M., *et al.* Zinc pre-treatment enhances NMDAR-mediated excitotoxicity in cultured cortical neurons from SOD1(G93A) mouse, a model of amyotrophic lateral sclerosis. *Neuropharmacology* 60, 1200-1208 (2011).
[135] Brunet, N., Tarabal, O., Esquerda, J.E. and Caldero, J. Excitotoxic motoneuron degeneration induced by glutamate receptor agonists and mitochondrial toxins in organotypic cultures of chick embryo spinal cord. *J. Comp. Neurol.*516, 277-290 (2009).
[136] Sasabe, J., *et al.* D-serine is a key determinant of glutamate toxicity in amyotrophic lateral sclerosis. *EMBO J.* 26, 4149-4159 (2007).
[137] Mitchell, J., *et al.* Familial amyotrophic lateral sclerosis is associated with a mutation in D-amino acid oxidase. *Proc. Natl. Acad. Sci. U S A*107, 7556-7561 (2010).
[138] Sasabe, J., *et al.* D-amino acid oxidase controls motoneuron degeneration through D-serine. *Proc. Natl. Acad. Sci. U S A*109, 627-632 (2012).
[139] Camacho, A. and Massieu, L. Role of glutamate transporters in the clearance and release of glutamate during ischemia and its relation to neuronal death. *Arch. Med. Res.* 37, 11-18 (2006).
[140] Doshi, S. and Lynch, D.R. Calpain and the glutamatergic synapse. *Front Biosci. (Schol Ed)*1, 466-476 (2009).
[141] Lau, A. and Tymianski, M. Glutamate receptors, neurotoxicity and neurodegeneration. *Pflugers. Arch.* 460, 525-542 (2010).
[142] Ono, Y. and Sorimachi, H. Calpains: an elaborate proteolytic system. *Biochim. Biophys. Acta* 1824, 224-236 (2012).
[143] Pivovarova, N.B. and Andrews, S.B. Calcium-dependent mitochondrial function and dysfunction in neurons. *FEBS J.* 277, 3622-3636 (2010).
[144] Shi, P., Wei, Y., Zhang, J., Gal, J. and Zhu, H. Mitochondrial dysfunction is a converging point of multiple pathological pathways in amyotrophic lateral sclerosis. *J. Alzheimers Dis.* 20 Suppl 2, S311-324 (2010).
[145] Brown, G.C. Nitric oxide and neuronal death. *Nitric. Oxide* 23, 153-165 (2010).
[146] Cao, J., *et al.* The PSD95-nNOS interface: a target for inhibition of excitotoxic p38 stress-activated protein kinase activation and cell death. *J. Cell Biol.* 168, 117-126 (2005).
[147] Wahl, A.S., *et al.* Hypoxic/ischemic conditions induce expression of the putative pro-death gene Clca1 via activation of extrasynaptic N-methyl-D-aspartate receptors. *Neuroscience*158, 344-352 (2009).
[148] Zhang, S.J., *et al.* Decoding NMDA receptor signaling: identification of genomic programs specifying neuronal survival and death. *Neuron* 53, 549-562 (2007).
[149] Espenshade, P.J. and Hughes, A.L. Regulation of sterol synthesis in eukaryotes. *Annu. Rev. Genet.* 41, 401-427 (2007).
[150] Goldstein, J.L., DeBose-Boyd, R.A. and Brown, M.S. Protein sensors for membrane sterols. *Cell* 124, 35-46 (2006).
[151] Yabe, D., Brown, M.S. and Goldstein, J.L. Insig-2, a second endoplasmic reticulum protein that binds SCAP and blocks export of sterol regulatory element-binding proteins. *Proc. Natl. Acad. Sci. U S A*99, 12753-12758 (2002).
[152] Jeon, T.I. and Osborne, T.F. SREBPs: metabolic integrators in physiology and metabolism. *Trends Endocrinol Metab*23, 65-72 (2012).

[153] McPherson, R. and Gauthier, A. Molecular regulation of SREBP function: the Insig-SCAP connection and isoform-specific modulation of lipid synthesis. *Biochem. Cell Biol.* 82, 201-211 (2004).

[154] St Pierre, P. and Nabi, I.R. The Gp78 ubiquitin ligase: probing endoplasmic reticulum complexity. *Protoplasma* 249 Suppl 1, S11-18 (2012).

[155] Bernasconi, R. and Molinari, M. ERAD and ERAD tuning: disposal of cargo and of ERAD regulators from the mammalian ER. *Curr. Opin. Cell Biol.* 23, 176-183 (2011).

[156] Smith, M.H., Ploegh, H.L. and Weissman, J.S. Road to ruin: targeting proteins for degradation in the endoplasmic reticulum. *Science* 334, 1086-1090 (2011).

[157] Gong, Y., *et al.* Sterol-regulated ubiquitination and degradation of Insig-1 creates a convergent mechanism for feedback control of cholesterol synthesis and uptake. *Cell Metab.* 3, 15-24 (2006).

[158] Lee, J.N., Gong, Y., Zhang, X. and Ye, J. Proteasomal degradation of ubiquitinated Insig proteins is determined by serine residues flanking ubiquitinated lysines. *Proc. Natl. Acad. Sci. U S A*103, 4958-4963 (2006).

[159] Lee, J.N., Song, B., DeBose-Boyd, R.A. and Ye, J. Sterol-regulated degradation of Insig-1 mediated by the membrane-bound ubiquitin ligase gp78. *J. Biol. Chem.* 281, 39308-39315 (2006).

[160] Ikeda, Y., *et al.* Regulated endoplasmic reticulum-associated degradation of a polytopic protein: p97 recruits proteasomes to Insig-1 before extraction from membranes. *J. Biol. Chem.* 284, 34889-34900 (2009).

[161] Lee, J.N., Zhang, X., Feramisco, J.D., Gong, Y. and Ye, J. Unsaturated fatty acids inhibit proteasomal degradation of Insig-1 at a postubiquitination step. *J. Biol. Chem.* 283, 33772-33783 (2008).

[162] Lee, J.N. and Ye, J. Proteolytic activation of sterol regulatory element-binding protein induced by cellular stress through depletion of Insig-1. *J. Biol. Chem.* 279, 45257-45265 (2004).

[163] Schwarze, S.R., Ho, A., Vocero-Akbani, A. and Dowdy, S.F. In vivo protein transduction: delivery of a biologically active protein into the mouse. *Science* 285, 1569-1572 (1999).

[164] Diraison, F., *et al.* SREBP1 is required for the induction by glucose of pancreatic beta-cell genes involved in glucose sensing. *J. Lipid. Res.* 49, 814-822 (2008).

[165] Sandberg, M.B., *et al.* Glucose-induced lipogenesis in pancreatic beta-cells is dependent on SREBP-1. *Mol. Cell Endocrinol.* 240, 94-106 (2005).

[166] Takahashi, A., *et al.* Transgenic mice overexpressing nuclear SREBP-1c in pancreatic beta-cells. *Diabetes* 54, 492-499 (2005).

[167] Wang, H., Kouri, G. and Wollheim, C.B. ER stress and SREBP-1 activation are implicated in beta-cell glucolipotoxicity. *J. Cell Sci.* 118, 3905-3915 (2005).

[168] Wang, H., *et al.* The transcription factor SREBP-1c is instrumental in the development of beta-cell dysfunction. *J. Biol. Chem.* 278, 16622-16629 (2003).

[169] Yamashita, T., *et al.* Role of uncoupling protein-2 up-regulation and triglyceride accumulation in impaired glucose-stimulated insulin secretion in a beta-cell lipotoxicity model overexpressing sterol regulatory element-binding protein-1c. *Endocrinology* 145, 3566-3577.

[170] Chang, Y.C., Bien, C.M., Lee, H., Espenshade, P.J. and Kwon-Chung, K.J. Sre1p, a regulator of oxygen sensing and sterol homeostasis, is required for virulence in Cryptococcus neoformans. *Mol. Microbiol.* 64, 614-629 (2007).

[171] Todd, B.L., Stewart, E.V., Burg, J.S., Hughes, A.L. and Espenshade, P.J. Sterol regulatory element binding protein is a principal regulator of anaerobic gene expression in fission yeast. *Mol. Cell Biol.* 26, 2817-2831 (2006).

[172] Powell-Coffman, J.A. Hypoxia signaling and resistance in C. elegans. *Trends Endocrinol. Metab.* 21, 435-440 (2010).

[173] Taghibiglou, C., *et al.* Essential role of SBP-1 activation in oxygen deprivation induced lipid accumulation and increase in body width/length ratio in Caenorhabditis elegans. *FEBS Lett.* 583, 831-834 (2009).

[174] Bien, C.M. and Espenshade, P.J. Sterol regulatory element binding proteins in fungi: hypoxic transcription factors linked to pathogenesis. *Eukaryot Cell*9, 352-359 (2010).

[175] Dahlman, I. and Arner, P. Genetics of adipose tissue biology. *Prog. Mol. Biol. Transl. Sci.* 94, 39-74 (2010).

[176] Raghow, R., Yellaturu, C., Deng, X., Park, E.A. and Elam, M.B. SREBPs: the crossroads of physiological and pathological lipid homeostasis. *Trends Endocrinol. Metab.*19, 65-73 (2008).

[177] Blum, R., *et al.* Molecular signatures of prostate stem cells reveal novel signaling pathways and provide insights into prostate cancer. *PLoS One* 4, e5722 (2009).

[178] Ettinger, S.L., *et al.* Dysregulation of sterol response element-binding proteins and downstream effectors in prostate cancer during progression to androgen independence. *Cancer Res.* 64, 2212-2221 (2004).

[179] Kuhajda, F.P. Fatty-acid synthase and human cancer: new perspectives on its role in tumor biology. *Nutrition* 16, 202-208 (2000).

[180] Liu, H., Liu, J.Y., Wu, X. and Zhang, J.T. Biochemistry, molecular biology, and pharmacology of fatty acid synthase, an emerging therapeutic target and diagnosis/prognosis marker. *Int. J. Biochem. Mol. Biol.* 1, 69-89 (2010).

[181] Plantier, L., *et al.* Activation of sterol-response element-binding proteins (SREBP) in alveolar type II cells enhances lipogenesis causing pulmonary lipotoxicity. *J. Biol. Chem.* 287, 10099-10114 (2012).

[182] Zhang, H.M., *et al.* Coxsackievirus B3 infection activates the unfolded protein response and induces apoptosis through downregulation of p58IPK and activation of CHOP and SREBP1. *J. Virol.* 84, 8446-8459 (2010).

[183] Del Campo, J.A. and Romero-Gomez, M. Steatosis and insulin resistance in hepatitis C: a way out for the virus? *World J. Gastroenterol.* 15, 5014-5019 (2009).

[184] Zager, R.A., Johnson, A., Anderson, K. and Wright, S. Cholesterol ester accumulation: an immediate consequence of acute in vivo ischemic renal injury. *Kidney Int.* 59, 1750-1761 (2001).

[185] Zager, R.A., Johnson, A.C. and Hanson, S.Y. Renal tubular triglyercide accumulation following endotoxic, toxic, and ischemic injury. *Kidney Int.* 67, 111-121 (2005).

[186] Zager, R.A., *et al.* The mevalonate pathway during acute tubular injury: selected determinants and consequences. *Am. J. Pathol.* 161, 681-692 (2002).

[187] Ruzzin, J., *et al.* Persistent organic pollutant exposure leads to insulin resistance syndrome. *Environ Health Perspect.* 118, 465-471 (2010).

[188] Caban-Holt, A., Mattingly, M., Cooper, G. and Schmitt, F.A. Neurodegenerative memory disorders: a potential role of environmental toxins. *Neurol. Clin.* 23, 485-521 (2005).

[189] Shaw, C.A. and Hoglinger, G.U. Neurodegenerative diseases: neurotoxins as sufficient etiologic agents? *Neuromolecular. Med.* 10, 1-9 (2008).

[190] Adibhatla, R.M. and Hatcher, J.F. Altered lipid metabolism in brain injury and disorders. *Subcell. Biochem.* 49, 241-268 (2008).

[191] Adibhatla, R.M. and Hatcher, J.F. Lipid oxidation and peroxidation in CNS health and disease: from molecular mechanisms to therapeutic opportunities. *Antioxid. Redox. Signal*12, 125-169 (2010).

[192] Bi, X. and Liao, G. Cholesterol in Niemann-Pick Type C disease. *Subcell. Biochem.* 51, 319-335 (2010).

[193] Dietschy, J.M. Central nervous system: cholesterol turnover, brain development and neurodegeneration. *Biol. Chem.* 390, 287-293 (2009).

[194] Florent-Bechard, S., *et al.* The essential role of lipids in Alzheimer's disease. *Biochimie.* 91, 804-809 (2009).

[195] Haughey, N.J. Sphingolipids in neurodegeneration. *Neuromolecular Med.* 12, 301-305 (2010).

[196] Haughey, N.J., Bandaru, V.V., Bae, M. and Mattson, M.P. Roles for dysfunctional sphingolipid metabolism in Alzheimer's disease neuropathogenesis. *Biochim. Biophys. Acta* 1801, 878-886 (2010).

[197] Ledesma, M.D. and Dotti, C.G. Peripheral cholesterol, metabolic disorders and Alzheimer's disease. *Front Biosci. (Elite Ed)*4, 181-194 (2012).

[198] Peake, K.B. and Vance, J.E. Defective cholesterol trafficking in Niemann-Pick C-deficient cells. *FEBS Lett.* 584, 2731-2739 (2010).

[199] Ruiperez, V., Darios, F. and Davletov, B. Alpha-synuclein, lipids and Parkinson's disease. *Prog. Lipid Res.* 49, 420-428 (2010).

[200] Schengrund, C.L. Lipid rafts: keys to neurodegeneration. *Brain Res. Bull.* 82, 7-17 (2010).

[201] Ferraiuolo, L., *et al.* Microarray analysis of the cellular pathways involved in the adaptation to and progression of motor neuron injury in the SOD1 G93A mouse model of familial ALS. *J. Neurosci.* 27, 9201-9219 (2007).

[202] Horton, J.D., *et al.* Combined analysis of oligonucleotide microarray data from transgenic and knockout mice identifies direct SREBP target genes. *Proc. Natl. Acad. Sci. U S A*100, 12027-12032 (2003).

[203] Park, H.J., *et al.* Role of sterol regulatory element binding proteins in the regulation of Galpha (i2) expression in cultured atrial cells. *Circ. Res.* 91, 32-37 (2002).

[204] Park, H.J., *et al.* Parasympathetic response in chick myocytes and mouse heart is controlled by SREBP. *J. Clin. Invest.* 118, 259-271 (2008).

[205] Reed, B.D., Charos, A.E., Szekely, A.M., Weissman, S.M. and Snyder, M. Genome-wide occupancy of SREBP1 and its partners NFY and SP1 reveals novel functional roles and combinatorial regulation of distinct classes of genes. *PLoS Genet.* 4, e1000133 (2008).

[206] Lewis, C.A., Griffiths, B., Santos, C.R., Pende, M. and Schulze, A. Regulation of the SREBP transcription factors by mTORC1. *Biochem. Soc. Trans.* 39, 495-499 (2011).

[207] Porstmann, T., *et al.* SREBP activity is regulated by mTORC1 and contributes to Akt-dependent cell growth. *Cell Metab*8, 224-236 (2008).
[208] Cleveland, D.W. and Rothstein, J.D. From Charcot to Lou Gehrig: deciphering selective motor neuron death in ALS. *Nat. Rev. Neurosci.* 2, 806-819 (2001).
[209] Oosthuyse, B., *et al.* Deletion of the hypoxia-response element in the vascular endothelial growth factor promoter causes motor neuron degeneration. *Nat. Genet.* 28, 131-138 (2001).
[210] Sebastia, J., *et al.* Angiogenin protects motoneurons against hypoxic injury. *Cell Death Differ.* 16, 1238-1247 (2009).
[211] Xu, R., *et al.* Linking hypoxic and oxidative insults to cell death mechanisms in models of ALS. *Brain Res.* 1372, 133-144 (2011).
[212] Zhong, Z., *et al.* ALS-causing SOD1 mutants generate vascular changes prior to motor neuron degeneration. *Nat. Neurosci.* 11, 420-422 (2008).
[213] Bergmann, F. and Keller, B.U. Impact of mitochondrial inhibition on excitability and cytosolic Ca2+ levels in brainstem motoneurones from mouse. *J. Physiol.* 555, 45-59 (2004).
[214] O'Reilly, J.P., Jiang, C. and Haddad, G.G. Major differences in response to graded hypoxia between hypoglossal and neocortical neurons. *Brain Res.* 683, 179-186 (1995).
[215] Kim, J.H., Jittiwat, J., Ong, W.Y., Farooqui, A.A. and Jenner, A.M. Changes in cholesterol biosynthetic and transport pathways after excitotoxicity. *J. Neurochem.* 112, 34-41 (2010).
[216] Ong, W.Y., *et al.* Changes in brain cholesterol metabolome after excitotoxicity. *Mol. Neurobiol.* 41, 299-313 (2010).
[217] Bjorkhem, I., *et al.* Cholesterol homeostasis in human brain: turnover of 24S-hydroxycholesterol and evidence for a cerebral origin of most of this oxysterol in the circulation. *J. Lipid Res.* 39, 1594-1600 (1998).
[218] Sodero, A.O., *et al.* Cholesterol loss during glutamate-mediated excitotoxicity. *EMBO J.* 31, 1764-1773 (2012).
[219] Bjorkhem, I. and Meaney, S. Brain cholesterol: long secret life behind a barrier. *Arterioscler Thromb. Vasc. Biol.* 24, 806-815 (2004).
[220] Thelen, K.M., Falkai, P., Bayer, T.A. and Lutjohann, D. Cholesterol synthesis rate in human hippocampus declines with aging. *Neurosci. Lett.* 403, 15-19 (2006).
[221] Fergani, A., *et al.* Increased peripheral lipid clearance in an animal model of amyotrophic lateral sclerosis. *J. Lipid Res.* 48, 1571-1580 (2007).
[222] Dupuis, L., *et al.* Dyslipidemia is a protective factor in amyotrophic lateral sclerosis. *Neurology* 70, 1004-1009 (2008).
[223] Dorst, J., *et al.* Patients with elevated triglyceride and cholesterol serum levels have a prolonged survival in amyotrophic lateral sclerosis. *J. Neurol.* 258, 613-617 (2011).
[224] Sutedja, N.A., *et al.* Beneficial vascular risk profile is associated with amyotrophic lateral sclerosis. *J. Neurol. Neurosurg. Psychiatry* 82, 638-642 (2011).
[225] Chio, A., *et al.* Lower serum lipid levels are related to respiratory impairment in patients with ALS. *Neurology* 73, 1681-1685 (2009).
[226] Kim, S.M., *et al.* Amyotrophic lateral sclerosis is associated with hypolipidemia at the presymptomatic stage in mice. *PLoS One*6, e17985 (2011).

[227] Patel, B.P., Safdar, A., Raha, S., Tarnopolsky, M.A. and Hamadeh, M.J. Caloric restriction shortens lifespan through an increase in lipid peroxidation, inflammation and apoptosis in the G93A mouse, an animal model of ALS. *PLoS One* 5, e9386 (2010).
[228] Park, K.G., *et al.* Alpha-lipoic acid decreases hepatic lipogenesis through adenosine monophosphate-activated protein kinase (AMPK)-dependent and AMPK-independent pathways. *Hepatology* 48, 1477-1486 (2008).
[229] Patel, B.P. and Hamadeh, M.J. Nutritional and exercise-based interventions in the treatment of amyotrophic lateral sclerosis. *Clin. Nutr.* 28, 604-617 (2009).
[230] Zinman, L., Sadeghi, R., Gawel, M., Patton, D. and Kiss, A. Are statin medications safe in patients with ALS? *Amyotroph. Lateral. Scler.* 9, 223-228 (2008).
[231] Golomb, B.A., Kwon, E.K., Koperski, S. and Evans, M.A. Amyotrophic lateral sclerosis-like conditions in possible association with cholesterol-lowering drugs: an analysis of patient reports to the University of California, San Diego (UCSD) Statin Effects Study. *Drug Saf.* 32, 649-661 (2009).

In: Amyotrophic Lateral Sclerosis
Editors: Katashi Segawa and Ryota Ijichi

ISBN: 978-1-62257-679-1

Chapter 3

Molecular Targeted Therapy against Amyotrophic Lateral Sclerosis

***Makoto Urushitani** *and Toshifumi Morimura*†**
Shiga University of Medical Science, Molecular Neuroscience Research Center,
Seta-Tsukinowa-cho, Otsu, Shiga, Japan

ABSTARCT

Abnormal deposition of ubiquitinated proteins is one of the key pathological features in various neurological disorders. The aggregates are composed of some "core proteins" that are unique to diseases. In amyotrophic lateral sclerosis (ALS), two major proteins have been intensively studied: one is mutant forms of superoxide dismutase 1 (SOD1) accounting for 20% of familial ALS; another is TAR DNA binding protein 43kDa (TDP-43), a central component of ubiquitinated inclusions of sporadic ALS patients. These proteins cause diverse pathogenic cascades both intra- and extra-cellular milieu, leading to motor neuron degeneration in ALS. In particular, recent lines of evidence imply that ALS-linked misfolded proteins could serve as seeds to nucleate their native forms, and even could be propagated from cell to cell. This scenario is attracting increasing attention as a potential mechanisms underlying irreversible disease progression. Therefore, a molecular targeting against such proteins both inside and outside motor neurons is a reasonable and practical approach for ALS. Target candidates vary in size from larger species such as oligomers, protofibrils, or aggregates, to specific amino acid residues of the protein. Accordingly, one of the aims of the molecular targeting is to trap or clear aberrantly assembled proteins. Another strategy is to attack pathogenic structures localized in disease-causal proteins to prevent further misfolding. The antibody medicine perfectly fits this end due to an advantage of the target-specific recognition. Either active or passive immunization against mutant SOD1 effectively expands the longevity of ALS model mice. Moreover, several murine monoclonal antibodies recognizing only misfolded SOD1 proteins, but not native forms, have been developed, and provided a therapeutic benefit on the mutant SOD1 transgenic mice. Furthermore, the recent advance in technology of antibody engineering allows us to transform monoclonal antibody of

* Email: uru@belle.shiga-med.ac.jp, TEL/Fax: +81-77-548-2328.
† Email: morimura@belle.shiga-med.ac.jp, TEL/Fax: +81-77-548-2402.

mouse-origin to humanized immunoglobulin or to generate a single chain of the fragment of variance (scFv) to be used for the intrabody. In addition, several small compounds are shown to prevent aggregation of mutant SOD1 or TDP-43, and high-throughput screening of more effective molecules is underway. To expand the potential of molecular targeted therapy, the structural analysis is expected for the identification of their pathogenic microdomains of ALS-linked proteins such as mutant SOD1 and TDP-43.

INTRODUCTION

A couple of decades ago, no one could have imagined that there are so diverse players and cascades involved in the pathogenesis of amyotrophic lateral sclerosis (ALS). ALS had been such a clueless disease despite the clear clinical and pathological features based on relatively selective motor neuron death[1]. This is chiefly because of limited information regarding on-going events in the nervous systems of ALS patients. However, researchers had struggled to develop experimental models for ALS to clarify the pathogenic cascades, including pharmacological settings using immortalized or primary culture cells from rodent embryos [2-5], and transgenic or knock-out animal models for ALS-linked proteins in the familial or sporadic ALS cases, such as mutant superoxide dismutase 1 (SOD1) and TAR DNA-binding protein 43 kDa (TDP-43) [6, 7]. These ALS models have informed us molecular pathways or machineries such as glutamate-induced excitotoxicity, mitochondrial dysfunction, oxidative stress, neuroinflammation, proteasome impairment, endoplasmic reticulum (ER) stress, axonal flow damage, protein misfolding, and abnormal RNA metabolisms [8-13]. Therefore, it is quite important to recognize that ALS is a multifactorial disorder; the conquest of ALS requires effective and simultaneous targeting strategies against 1) specific key molecules involved in the pathogenesis, 2) general events, including calcium influx, oxidative stress, and neuroinflammation, and 3) affected organelles such as mitochondria and ER.

So far, the only FDA-approved medication is riluzole, a presynaptic glutamate release inhibitor [14-16]. This is based on the experimental evidence that the glutamate transport is affected due to the selective reduction of a glial transporter (EAAT2 or GLT1) in the brain and spinal cord tissues from ALS patients [17, 18]. Ceaseless attempts for drug screening to modulate EAAT2 are underway; as one candidate, ceftriaxone is now tested in the clinical trial in the U.S.A. Although many attempts to detoxify oxidative stress, to improve mitochondrial functions, or to promote regeneration of motor neurons unfortunately have ended up with discouraging outcomes [19-21], newly developed chemical, KNS760704, a mitochondrial modulator, brought about promising effect in the clinical trials for ALS [22].

Another important clue to understand ALS is an aberrant conformational change of ALS-linked proteins. Foresighted neuropathological investigations by many frontiers have identified unique cytoplasmic inclusions in the affected regions of sporadic [23-25] or familial [24, 26] ALS patients, including skein-like and Lewy body-like hyaline inclusions. There is a growing consensus that mutant SOD1 and TDP-43 are among pathogenic core proteins of these inclusions in familial and sporadic ALS, respectively. Although the exact pathogenesis how these proteins cause ALS remains unclear, they are undoubtedly definite triggers for many noxious cascades as mentioned above. In particular, it is a current consensus that protein misfolding underlies the molecular transformation to oligomers and aggregates, which are supposed to play key roles in neurodegeneration. Based on this knowledge, a growing attention has been paid to the therapeutic strategies aiming to manipulate such aberrant proteins. The most target-specific medication is an antibody. Precedent works on Alzheimer's disease targeting detrimental amyloid-β proteins by the vaccination have demonstrated a significant benefit to clear senile plaques in the brain of patients with Alzheimer's disease [27]. Moreover, various monoclonal antibodies recognizing specific epitopes have been developed. Unfortunately, the clinical outcome of the immunization in Alzheimer's disease is somewhat discouraging, because of the serious adverse reactions or limited benefit to prevent the cognitive decline [27]. However, one interpretation is that the amyloid aggregates are not dominant executors for neurodegeneration; another explanation is participation of other proteins such as phosphorylated-tau, which is also to be targeted. On the other hand, there is no doubt as to the central roles of mutant SOD1 and TDP-43 in the pathogenesis in ALS, which may well justify the targeting therapy against them.

Intriguingly, accumulating evidence indicates that disease-causal proteins, including α-synuclein, huntingtin, phosphorylated tau, and mutant SOD1 could be transmitted to the neighboring cells, as if they were prion proteins. This "prionoid" behavior of various disease-linked proteins could explain how affected lesions gradually widen along with the neurodegeneration. These backgrounds prompt us to focus on the active or passive immunization against the causal misfolded proteins in ALS, as well as in various neurodegenerative diseases.

This chapter first illustrates molecular backgrounds how ALS-linked proteins are transformed to the misfolded and toxic forms. Later, the current progress in the research of the molecular targeted therapy, especially against mutant SOD1 and TDP-43 will be presented.

Abnormal Inclusions and Protein Misfolding

Protein turnover is a fundamental determinant for cellular homeostasis. During the synthesis, proteins are to be properly folded to form the strictly defined conformation. Protein folding is regulated by intramolecular associations such as disulfide and hydrogen bonds, and the help of molecular chaperons, including heat shock protein is required. However, amino acid substitutions due to the genetic mutations resulted in the altered folding patterns, especially in the intramolecular associations, which lead to aberrant conformation, so-called misfolded proteins. Moreover, the role of molecular chaperons becomes more important to refold the misfolded proteins, which accounts for pathological features that abnormal inclusions are often Hsp70-positive [28, 29]. A crucial cellular defense mechanism to protect cells from detrimental events caused by misfolded proteins is a ubiquitin-proteasome system (UPS). UPS consists of three molecules, ubiquitin activating enzyme (E1), ubiquitin converting enzyme (E2) and ubiquitin ligase (E3). Through the effect of the ensemble of these enzymes, target proteins are conjugated with poly-ubiquitin chains. Poly-ubiquitinated proteins are transferred to the protein degradation machinery, called proteasome, where proteins are digested into small peptide fragments by several enzymes, such as tryptic, chymotryptic, and PGDH-like proteases. For instance, mutant SOD1 proteins are recognized by UPS as aberrant protein products. Therefore, their half-life is shorter than WT SOD1, since they are degraded at proteasomes so far as not to exceed its clearance capacity. Lysosome-dependent macroautophagy (referred to autophagy in this chapter) is another important elimination pathway of mutant SOD1 proteins [30]. It is shown that activation of autophagy not only enhances removal of mutant SOD1 but also prolongs life span of ALS model mice with a SOD1 mutation [31]. However, perpetual expression of mutant SOD1 impairs proteasome [32], and autophagy-mediated degradation [31], leading to the accumulation of undesirable proteins, including mutant SOD1 proteins themselves. Thus, the impairment of proteasome and autophagy are ranked high as causes of neurodegeneration. A molecular basis being postulated to transform misfolded proteins to the executors of cell death is a β-sheet. β-sheet conversion is required for prion proteins to acquire the toxic property as prion seeds. In Alzheimer's disease, β-sheet is a molecular signature of senile plaque. In Parkinson's disease, it is assumed that the initial β-sheet formation of α-synuclein monomer leads to toxic oligomer, protofibrils, and fibrils [33].

Interestingly, such as misfolded proteins are recognized as unusual pathogens beyond immunological tolerance, despite that they are originated from endogenous proteins. For instance, the vaccination using amyloid-β aggregates induce the high titration of antibody in both mice [34] and human [35]. Other than the aggregate forms, the monomeric conformer can also be an immunogen, including mutant α–synuclein or SOD1 against the model mice of Parkinson's disease [36] or ALS ([37, 38], respectively.

Collectively, it should be noted that disease-causal proteins are "pathogens" due to the aberrant structures compared with the native form.

Table 1. Identified or locus-specified genes for familial ALS

ALS disease types	chromosome	Gene	Gene symbol	Inheritance	Aggregate formation
ALS1	21q22.1	**superoxide dismutase 1**	**SOD1**	AD	yes
ALS2	2q33	amyotrophic laterals slerosis 2	ALS2	AR	no
ALS3	18q21	unknown	-	AD	
ALS4	9q34	senataxin	SETX	AD	NE
ALS5	15q15.1-21.1	unknown	-		
ALS6	16q12	Fused in sarcoma	FUS	AD/AR	yes
ALS7	20p13	unknown	-	AD	
ALS8	20q13.33	vesicle-associated membrane protein-associated protein B	VAPB	AD	yes
ALS9	14q11	angiogenin	ANG	AD	no
ALS10	1p36.22	**TAR DNA-binding protein**	**TARDBP**	AD	yes
ALS11	6q21	FIG4 homolog, SAC1 lipid phosphatase domain containing (S. cerevisiae)	FIG4	AR	NE
ALS12	10p13	optineurin	OPTN	AR/AD	yes

NE, not evaluated.

ALS-LINKED MISFOLDED PROTEINS

Increasing number of ALS-linked proteins have been unraveled. Most of these are products of mutant genes found in familial ALS cases (Table 1). So far, mutant SOD1, TDP-

43, and Fused in sarcoma (FUS) are among the most characterized proteins. They are detected as ubiquitin-positive inclusions in the affected regions, indicating that these proteins are recognized as aberrant proteins in the protein quality control system.

1. Superoxide Dismutase 1 (SOD1)

SOD1 was the first genetic mutation found in the subpopulation of familial ALS (FALS) patients [39]. SOD1 is a cytosolic metalloenzyme, which catalyzes superoxide anion to hydrogen peroxide and oxygen. Since the oxidative stress has been implicated in the major cause of various neurological diseases, the loss of SOD1 enzymatic activity was assumed to be a cause of ALS. However, results from several studies have argued against this hypothesis. First, knockout mice for SOD1 showed no phenotype of ALS [40] (This does not necessarily mean "no phenotype". They are indeed very sick). Second, although there are more than 100 mutations with different antioxidant activity, disease severity of ALS symptoms does not correlate to the antioxidant activity of SOD1. Third, transgenic mice expressing enzymatically inactive mutant SOD1 develop ALS [41]. Based on these results, our consensus is that mutant SOD1-linked ALS is mediated by toxic cascades based on the abnormal conformation, but not on the antioxidant property of SOD1.

SOD1 is a dimeric protein comprising Cu- and Zn-incorporated monomer. In spite of its location in the cytosol, a reducing environment, SOD1 monomer has an intramolecular disulfide bond; this linkage is quite important to maintain the metal incorporation and the proper dimer conformation. Therefore, it is plausible that a single amino acid substitution in any region of SOD1 may affect monomer conformation, resulting in exposing cysteine residues to the reductive environment of cytoplasm. However, the molecular basis of the misfolding mechanisms of SOD1 is complicated, since there are more than 100 types of mutations in various domains in SOD1. According to previous papers, these mutations can be classified into several groups depending on the susceptibility to the reducing agents [42] or the location of the protease-resistant regions [43]. These abnormal conformations may trigger various detrimental pathways by the interaction with unusual molecules, inducing additional chemical reactions or the subcellular mislocalizations.

1.1. In-Cell Pathomechanisms Caused by Mutant SOD1

There are diverse pathways caused by mutant SOD1 proteins, including excitotoxicity, proteasome impairment, mitochondrial dysfunction, oxidative stress, axonal flow damage, endoplasmic reticulum (ER) stress, and aggregation toxicity [8, 10, 12, 44]. Several molecules have been shown to interact with mutant SOD1, resulting in the aberrant subcellular localization. For instance, VDAC1 translocates mutant SOD1 to mitochondria [45], Bip or Derlin-1 does to ER [46, 47], so do chromogranins to trans-Golgi network [48]. These multiple binding partners may contribute to complicated pathways caused by mutant SOD1. To interpret the pathogenesis of ALS, the involvement of other cells than motor neurons should also be noted. In particular, microglial and astroglial cells play important roles to modulate development and progression of ALS. In contrast to numerous papers investigating the toxic cascades in motor neurons, limited information is available as to the *in-cell* event in glial cells expressing mutant SOD1. It is documented that primary cultured microglial cells displayed reduced expression of cell adhesion molecule, integrin beta-1.

However, there is no difference between WT and mutant SOD1 overexpression microglial cells in the phagocytosis, migration, and intracellular calcium release, which are more affected than in non-transgenic cells [49]. cDNA microarray analysis of primary astrocytes revealed the alteration of gene expression of transcription, signaling, cell proliferation, extracellular matrix synthesis, response to stress, and steroid and lipid metabolism [50]. Moreover, another study demonstrated various proinflammatory molecules, including prostaglandin D2 (PGD2) receptor, Monocyte Chemoattractant Protein 2 (MCP2), Chemokine (C-X-C motif) ligand 7 (CXCL7), and phagocytic NADPH oxidase (NOX2) [51]. However, overexpression of mutant SOD1 gene in a single cell-type in mice spinal cords does not cause ALS phenotype [52-55]. Therefore, mutant SOD1-linked ALS is non-cell-autonomous. This notion is quite important, since it expanded the therapeutic windows of ALS, and directed our eyes to the extracellular environment as a target.

1.2. Non-Cell-Autonomy of ALS Pathogenesis

Based on the previous transgenic findings, four major research groups in the USA and Canada tied up together to answer the question "Is mutant SOD1-linked ALS is really non-cell-autonomous?". A historical paper called "chimeric mice work" came out in 2003, documenting that motor neuron degeneration is not caused by the mutant proteins in the motor neurons, but by those in the surrounding cells such as microglia and astrocytes. Notably, the larger the number of neighboring cells expressing mutant SOD1, the severer the motor neuron damage is [56]. Later intensive investigation by the leading group using sophisticated approach called Cre-LoxP system, confirmed us this notion. From the observation of transgenic mice, lacking mutant SOD1 either in microglia, astrocytes, or in the motor neurons, it was clearly shown that the knockdown of motor neuronal SOD1 mutants delayed the onset of paralysis, whereas that of glial cells prolonged the disease progression with no influence on the onset [57, 58]. These results have made us to re-realize the non-cell-autonomy of mutant SOD1-linked ALS. More importantly, growing attention has been paid to astrocytes as crucial executors of motor neuron death. This notion is strongly supported by the evidence that nontransgenic motor neurons are killed by transgenic astrocytes expressing mutant SOD1 in cell culture study [59] and animal experiment [60]. However, a caution must be taken to interpret the ALS pathogenesis, since there is a report documenting cell-autonomous development of motor neuron death in mice [61]. Moreover, the effect to delay the onset or progression of ALS symptoms may be affected by the line of transgenic mice [62].

1.3. Extracellular Hypothesis and Protein Propagation Theory

After the notion of non-cell-autonomy of motor neuron death caused by mutant SOD1, the molecular hunting has enthusiastically been underway. Responsible molecules are assumed to mediate the crosstalk between neurons and glial cells, and even T lymphocytes as recently suggested [63]. Major players to link neurons and glial cells are proinflammatory molecules, which are expressed in astrocytes or microglia as described above. Matrix metalloproteinase 9 (MMP9), reportedly upregulated in both motor neurons and glial cells, induces tumor necrosis factor α (TNFα) and Fas ligand. Knockout of MMP9 from mutant SOD1 transgenic mice prominently extended the lifespan [64], indicating that MMP9 is one of the major modifiers of ALS pathogenesis. So far, proinflammatory molecules are recognized as potential targets of non-cell-autonomous motor neuron degeneration in ALS. On the other hand, the transgenic works describing the negative effect of astrocyte- or microglia-targeted overexpression of mutant SOD1 indicate that inflammation does not suffice to explain the development of ALS. We successfully identified a neurosecretory protein, chromogranin B, as an interacting partner with mutant SOD1, but not with the WT. Chromogranin B (ChgB) and its granin family member chromogranin A (ChgA), promote the secretion of mutant SOD1. Moreover, mutant SOD1 secreted or applied in the medium activates microglia and injures motor neurons [48]. Furthermore, chromogranin B was reported to be a risk factor in ALS [65]. The neurotoxicity of extracellular SOD1 mutants is in part mediated by microglial CD14, a glycoprotein functioning as a receptor for lipopolysaccharide (LPS) [66]. Interaction of mutant SOD1 and chromogranins are confirmed in the spinal cords of FALS patients (67). SOD1 proteins of mutant and WT are detected in the cerebrospinal fluid of ALS patients [68]. The overexpression of ChgA in the motor neurons of mutant SOD1 transgenic mice accelerated the onset of the paralysis [69].

Accumulating evidence indicates that mutant SOD1 proteins are transmitted to neighboring cells, not only secreted from cells [70-72]. Importantly, transmitted misfolded SOD1 proteins induce conversion of the native SOD1 to the misfolded species, which further promotes the spreading of misfolded SOD1 proteins. Grad et al. specified the tryptophan residues at the position of 32 amino acids as a responsible residue which mediates this conversion [72]. This prion-like behavior of mutant SOD1 should be further investigated if it is a dominant mechanism of the irreversible progression of neurodegeneration of mutant SOD1-linked FALS.

Collectively, evidence that mutant SOD1 can propagate to neighboring cells has cast new light on the molecular targeted therapy to capture extracellular mutant SOD1 proteins, as is proved by the success of vaccination or antibody therapy against mutant SOD1 proteins in ALS model mice [37, 73].

1.4. Misfolded SOD1 in Sporadic ALS

SOD1 is abundantly expressed in the cytoplasm, comprising two percentages of total cytosolic proteins. Therefore, it is no surprise that deformity of SOD1 causes detrimental effects on the cell viability. Indeed, wild-type SOD1 proteins subjected to oxidative modification or metal deprivation acquires the similar chemical properties of mutant SOD1, including ubiquitination, oligomerization, and interaction with heat-shock chaperones [29, 69, 74]. It should be noted that SOD1 aggregates are detected in the motor neurons in sporadic ALS patients [75]. Gruzman et al. demonstrated that aberrant dimer of SOD1 is a common biochemical feature shared in sporadic and mutant SOD1-linked ALS patients [76]. Surprisingly, it is reported that motor neurons of sporadic ALS patients contain oxidized SOD1 proteins, which are labeled by the monoclonal antibody against misfolded SOD1 (C4F6) [77], being raised against a specific type of mutant SOD1 [37]. Moreover, another report shows that ablation of SOD1 from cultured astrocytes obtained from sporadic ALS patients, prevents co-cultured motor neuron from astrocytes-mediated toxicity [78]. On the other hand, some reports argue against the involvement of WT SOD1 in sporadic ALS cases based on the failure to prove the presence of SOD1 in the spinal cord or CSF, using antibodies against misfolded SOD1[79, 80]. Nevertheless, it is our consensus that WT SOD1 acquires mutant-like molecular deformity, especially by the oxidation or metal-deprivation. However, the active role of misfolded SOD1 in sporadic ALS remains undetermined.

Therefore, the intensive research should be addressed to this issue, since this might give rise to another therapeutic option as a molecular target for sporadic ALS patients.

2. TAR DNA-Binding Protein 43 Kda (TDP-43)

TDP-43 was identified as a core of ubiquitinated inclusions in the brain of frontotemporal lobar degeneration (FTLD) through the mass-spectrometric analysis [81, 82]. While various proteins have been proposed as components of ubiquitinated inclusions in sporadic ALS, TDP-43 is quite frequently detected in sporadic or mutant SOD1-irrelevant ALS. TDP-43 is a DNA/RNA-binding protein with various functions, including RNA splicing, DNA/RNA stabilization, and microRNA metabolism. TDP-43 is composed of nucleus localizing signal (NLS), two RNA-binding domains (RRM1 and RRM2), and carboxyl tail containing glycine-rich domains. Nucleus export signal (NES) is located in the RRM2 domain. Neuropathological features of TDP-43 proteinopathy in ALS patients are relatively clear. Affected motor neurons lose nuclear TDP-43, accompanied by the mislocalization of TDP-43 in the cytosol. It is assumed that cytosolic TDP-43 proteins distribute homogenously in the initial phase, and later form inclusions such as skeins or Lewy body-like hyaline inclusions, which were frequently phosphorylated or ubiquitinated [83, 84]. Moreover, genetic mutations in TDP-43 have been identified in fractions of familial ALS patients [85-90], indicating its primary role in ALS pathogenesis.

2.1. Expression Levels and Subcellular Localization of TDP-43 in ALS Pathogenesis

Mice completely lacking TDP-43 are embryonic lethal [91], while postnatal knocking out of TDP-43 induces a rapid death with severe reduction of body lipid [92]. On the other hand, the transgenic mice overexpressing either mutant or wild-type TDP-43 display partial ALS phenotypes, including, motor impairment and cognitive disturbance [93-100]. Interestingly, cytosolic mislocalization of TDP-43 in motor neurons is not an early event in these mice, except one line carrying genome expression cassette for human TDP-43 [94]. Recent consensus is that TDP-43 proteinopathy is mediated by both loss of function of nuclear TDP-43 and gain of toxic functions of misfolded TDP-43. The loss of function hypothesis is well accepted, since it is clearly documented that nuclear TDP-43 is sequestered to cytosolic TDP-43 aggregates. The pathological evidence of the loss of nuclear TDP-43 staining in the affected regions in ALS patients supports this notion. Conversely, limited evidence is available as to the increase in TDP-43 in the affected regions. There is only one report demonstrating that TDP-43 in the spinal cord lysates from sporadic ALS patients is upregulated by two folds [101]. Taken together, it is plausible to assume that there are two critical stages for TDP-43 proteinopathy; first, nuclear upregulation, and second, the cytosolic redistribution.

2.2. Proposed Molecules Mediating TDP-43 Proteinopathy

In this chapter, we are focusing on the molecular targeted therapy in ALS. Unfortunately, however, information as to the toxic counterpart of TDP-43 is limited. TDP-43 has three groups of amino acid residues similar to the caspase recognition sequences [102]. In particular, the cleavage sites are located at the carboxyl side of NLS, and thus the cleaved products are transferred to the cytosol. Very interestingly, these products are same size to the TDP-43 fragments frequently detected in the tissue lysates of ALS or FTLD. Another TDP-43-binding protein is P65, a component of nuclear factor kappa B (NF-κB). NF-κB was identified in the lipopolysaccharide (LPS)-stimulated microglial cell-line and its transcriptional activity was enhanced by TDP43, indicating that TDP-43 is involved in the neuroinflammation. This notion is validated by the therapeutic benefit of Withaferin A, a potent NF-κB inhibitor to delay the progression of TDP-43 transgenic mice [101]. Fused in sarcoma (FUS) is also a well-known binding partner with TDP-43 [103]. However, molecular mechanisms how FUS/TDP-43 complex or disassembly exerts neurotoxicity is unknown. By the comprehensive approach of TDP-43-knockout cells to search for molecules with altered expression levels, several molecules have been identified, including the upregulation of cyclin-dependent kinase 6 [104], and the downregulation of histone deacetylase 6 (HDAC6)(105), and inactivation of the Rho family members RhoA, Rac1, and Cdc42 GTPases [106]. It is also reported that the knockdown of TDP-43 induces abnormal regulation of various micro RNA, which results in the affected the transcription of some candidate molecules responsible for TDP-43 proteinopathy [107].

2.3. Misfolded TDP-43 as a Therapeutic Target

TDP-43 is a RNA/DNA-interacting protein, the defect of which may well induce serious cell damage. Indeed, a huge number of RNAs have been identified to be processed by TDP-43 [108-110]. This means that TDP-43-related cascades are too numerous to prioritize a specific cascade as a therapeutic target. Therefore, increasing attention has been paid to identify intramolecular domains of TDP-43, which play important role in the protein misfolding. C-terminus of TDP-43 has been recognized as predominant target domain. The concentration of genetic mutations of TDP-43 in familial ALS patients, also signify the role of this fragments. Current research has uncovered increasing number of potentially pathogenic domains, which might mediate the misfolding of TDP-43 has been reported (described later).

3. Other ALS-Linked Misfolded Proteins

Fused in sarcoma (FUS): FUS is also a DNA/RNA-binding protein, the genetic mutations of which were found in the subpopulation of familial ALS patients. FUS has a similar domain structure as that of TDP-43. However, Mutant FUS-linked ALS shows an early onset and a rapid progression with basophilic inclusions in the remaining motor neurons, which is distinct from mutant TDP-43-linked ALS [111]. Transgenic rat for FUS of FALS-linked mutant, but not wild-type develop motor impairment and cognitive disturbance, mimicking ALS and frontotemporal lobar degeneration [111]. Pathomechanisms of FUS-induced ALS are under investigation.

Optineurin: It has been recognized that optineurin is a responsible gene for glaucoma [112]. Unexpectedly, genetic mutations in optineurin were identified in Japanese families with ALS, the locations of which differ from those of glaucoma [113]. Mode of inheritance is autosomal recessive or dominant. Optineurin mutations are relatively rare as shown in studies from in North America, Australia [114] and France [115]. However, it is noteworthy that optineurin is an autophagic adaptor ubiquitin binding protein [116], and it colocalized either with mutant SOD1 or with TDP-43 aggregates in ALS specimen, implying its involvement in the common pathway of ALS pathogenesis. More importantly, it is shown that optineurin represses the NFκB activity, leading to the inhibition of neuroinflammation [113]. However, evidence is not enough to discuss their potential as candidates for molecular targeted therapy.

MOLECULAR TARGETING: STRATEGY VIEW

Undoubtedly, neurodegeneration is caused by the combination of diverse *in-cell* and extracellular pathways. Therefore, the prioritization of the predominant cascade is ideal. However, it is practically difficult, due to quite many cascades, and to unexpected compensatory reactions induced by the blockade of specific molecules. Moreover, it should be noted that these diverse cascades were mostly downstream of protein misfolding of causal proteins. Furthermore, mounting evidence implies that misfolded proteins might spread and propagate to neighboring cells, which could underlie the progression of neurodegeneration. In this sense, causal proteins, mutant SOD1 and TDP-43 for ALS for instance, are promising therapeutic targets.

Molecular targeting therapy for ALS-linked misfolded proteins may comprise several strategies such as 1) the inhibition of synthesis, 2) enhancement of degradation, 3) the elimination by acquired immunity, and 4) domain attacking by small molecules or antibodies.

1. The Inhibition of Protein Synthesis

This can be applied to the mutant proteins, the expression of which is proven to be pathogenic, such as mutant SOD1 proteins. RNA silencing by small interference RNA (siRNA) is a strong tool to confer mutant-specific blockade of protein synthesis by an appropriated designing of nucleotides, so as not to affect the expression of wild-type proteins. The beneficial effect of RNA silencing against mutant SOD1 have been documented in the transgenic mice, in which lenti virus for siRNA (modified to continuously expressing shRNA) was injected into skeletal muscles [117] or spinal cords [118]. Although the effective gene silencing therapy basically requires the virus introduction, intraventricular infusion of anti-sense oligonucleotides provided a considerable effect to inhibit the expression of mutant SOD1 in the central nervous system [119]. It is also shown that external oligonucleotides effectively incorporated into glial cells s [119]. This experimental evidence allowed its clinical trial, currently underway. However, a drastic improvement of drug-delivery systems is inevitable, to target affected regions to augment the therapeutic effect.

In case of TDP-43, there is no report to document the effect of RNA silencing for the WT or mutant TDP-43 in the transgenic mice. Given that the mechanisms how WT/mutant TDP-43 provides motor neuron death in ALS remains unsolved, it is too early to consider RNA silencing as a therapeutic option.

2. Facilitation of Protein Degradation

Mutant SOD1 proteins are more unstable with shorter half-life than the WT [120]. This is because mutant proteins are misfolded and recognized by ubiquitin-proteasome system (UPS) [32]. UPS consists of ubiquitin activating enzyme (E1), ubiquitin converting enzyme (E2), and ubiquitin ligase (E3). E3 is a substrate-specific, although there is some redundancy. For instance, three kinds of ubiquitin ligase are reported to ubiquitinate mutant SOD1, including Dorfin [121], CHIP [29], and NEDL1 [122]. Double transgenic mice of mutant SOD1 and Dorfin showed an extended longevity significantly [123]. Surprisingly, however, NEDL1 transgenic mice develop ALS phenotype even in the absence of mutant SOD1, warning us the complexities of utilization of E3 as a therapy [124]. On the other hand, it is reported that mutant SOD1 is degraded by autophagy not only in proteasomes [30]. Proteolysis of TDP-43 also occurred at both proteasomes and autophagosomes [125]. Since the autophagy is basically a non-specific bulk-system for the clearance of organelles and aggregates, caution should be provided not to affect other physiological events by the gross enhancement of autophagy, as evidenced in the animal experiment, in which rapamycin failed to improve the progression of the paralysis [126]. It should be noted, however, the inhibitory effect of rapamycin on the activity of mammalian target of rapamycin (mTOR), required for the augmentation of autophagy, is partial [127]. Therefore, other potential compounds such as Trin1 and Trin2 [128] should be also tested in ALS model animals.

3. Scavenge of the Target Proteins by Acquired Immunity

It was a big surprise when a report demonstrating the effect of vaccination against amyloid-β in mice came out [34]. This pioneering work has been a followed by a huge number of experiments, and has reached clinical trials, although the outcome is not satisfactory [27]. The effective induction of antibodies against target proteins implies that misfolded proteins such as aggregates and oligomers have quite distinct conformations so as to be recognized by the acquired immunity. In ALS, vaccination (active immunization) against recombinant mutant SOD1 proteins purified from *E. coli* significantly extended the lifespan of ALS model mice (G37R) which have five-time higher levels of SOD1 expression compared with the endogenous SOD1. However, the same vaccination was unsuccessful in the high-copy ALS model mice expressing seventeen-time higher SOD1 proteins because of over an overwhelming expression level of mutant proteins to be scavenged by induced antibody [37]. This notion is supported by the therapeutic benefit of passive immunization, in which intraventricular infusion of affinity-purified antisera [37] or monoclonal antibodies [73] delayed the progression of ALS model mice. Remarkably, the intrathecal monoclonal antibody against mutant SOD1 decreases the amount of misfolded species of the mutant SOD1 protein in the spinal cord [73]. Recent evidence has highlighted the involvement of misfolded form of WT SOD1 in the pathogenesis of sporadic ALS [75-77]. Experimentally, the metal-deprivation or the oxidative modification of WT SOD1 induces its misfolding [29, 69]. Indeed, the vaccination with misfolded WT SOD1 protein (demetallated) significantly extends the longevity of mutant SOD1 transgenic mice [38]. Mechanisms how the immunization confers the neuroprotection have been a mystery. However, accumulating evidence has convinced us that mutant SOD1 proteins are secreted and propagated into neighboring cells [48, 70, 72]. Therefore, it is plausible that antibody targets extracellular SOD1 mutant proteins to prevent their effect on the microglial activation or propagation.

In the case of TDP-43, the research is enthusiastically ongoing on their prionoid behaviors. So far, however, no compelling evidence has been provided.

4. Attacking of Pathogenic Domains in the Target Molecule

Pathogenic domains in this chapter refer to the specific amino acid residues, which physically associate with other molecules such as receptors, or are involved in the protein misfolding. In mutant SOD1, several candidate sequences have been proposed. For instance, cysteine at 57 and 146 of SOD1 are shown to mediate the formation of disulfide-mediated oligomers [129]. Other papers have documented the role of cysteine 111 in oligomerization of SOD1 [130, 131]. Strikingly, the mass-spectrometric (MS/MS) analysis of immune-precipitates with antibody against P2X4, a subunit of ATP receptor, turned out to be fragments of SOD1 mutant proteins (Ser34 to His51). Moreover, parenchymal infusion of this fragment, but not WT-derived species robustly induced microglial activation [132]. A structural approach using nuclear magnetic resonance (NMR) uncovered unstable residues at Ala60, Gly61, Pro62, His63, and Phe64 during the early misfolding of mutant SOD1 proteins [133]. Another approach using MS/MS analysis of aggregated species of recombinant SOD1 proteins unraveled several aggregation cores that were undigested by protease [43]. It was shown that monoclonal antibody against misfolded SOD1 (D3H5) provided the same therapeutic effect in either form of full-length IgG or of Fab fragments [73]. This clearly indicates that D3H5 monoclonal antibody neutralizes mutant SOD1 by attacking the specific residues that confer the toxicity.

As a molecular targeting tool, small compounds are quite promising. By using reliable *in vitro* models or cell culture systems mimicking ALS, dozens of chemicals can be screened whether they can prevent aggregate formation in these models. For instance, cyclohexane 1,3-diones (CHD) derivatives were identified from high throughput screening for aggregate prevention in transfected cultured cells (PC12 cells) expressing fluorescent mutant SOD1 proteins [134]. Notably, these compounds have different effects depending on the cell types, and the beneficial effect to prolong the longevity of mutant SOD1 transgenic mice is not remarkable. Further modification of the compounds to improve the delivery to central nervous system, or membrane permeability may ameliorate the effect. Another interesting strategy is to screen small compounds targeting the promoter for molecule-specific transcription[135].

In TDP-43, growing evidence demonstrates specific amino acid residues or peptides sequences, which may regulate the protein folding. For instance, MS/MS analysis of undigested fragments of protease-treated TDP-43 revealed that protease-resistant peptides are concentrated at carboxyl terminus and the region of the RRM1-RRM2 transition [136]. The other candidate domains are cysteine residues, presumably involved in the disulfide-mediated oligomer formation [137].

Considering that most of the misfolded proteins are originated from endogenous proteins, the whole clearance or knockdown strategy might not be practical approaches. Rather, recognition and attacking of pathogenic regions are desirable. In this sense, structural analysis of disease causal proteins such as NMR, X-ray crystal and modified proteomics approaches, will be more and more important.

MOLECULAR TARGETING USING ANTIBODY MEDICINE

In terms of target-specific reaction, antibody is an ideal therapeutic tool. Above all, monoclonal antibodies have a huge potential in terms of their diverse applications in pharmacology and molecular biology. Immunoglobulin comprises the variable region (VL) and constant region. VL contains antigen binding domains, called complementarity determining region (CDR). The amino acid sequence of the constant region is species-specific, which is to be replaced to the humane one for the clinical use (chimeric immunoglobulin). Recently, a complete humanization of mice-derived monoclonal antibody has been available, in which other regions than CDR are totally replaced to the residues of human IgG. In light of recent development of various monoclonal antibodies against misfolded SOD1 proteins, together with the notion that mutant SOD1 protein could propagate to neighboring cells(37, 72, 73), passive immunization using humanized version of these monoclonal antibodies is expected as a promising therapy to halt the disease progression.

Another useful application of monoclonal antibody is a single chain of variable fragment (scFv), which can be obtained from messenger RNA of hybridoma cells or phage library. scFv is usually made from tandem VH and VL proteins, in which flexible hinge on peptides link them to mimic antigen binding region of immunoglobulin. VH or VL fragment alone can also be available depending on the antibody. Intrabody refers to scFv, which is designed to express inside cells using mammalian expression vectors. In cell culture studies, it is successfully shown that intrabodies recognize and diminish aggregated huntingtin [138] or αsynuclein [138]. Strikingly, intramuscular delivery of scFv against amyloid β protein by virus vector prevents deposition of amyloid plaques and ameliorates the cognitive decline of Alzheimer model mice [139].

In addition, monoclonal antibodies have many other applications, including high throughput screening of chemical compounds, which competes with the antibodies to interact with the same epitope domains.

FUTURE PERSPECTIVES OF MOLECULAR TARGETING THERAPY

In light of the recent consensus that misfolded forms of disease-causal proteins play a primary role in the neurodegeneration, molecular targeted therapy against such proteins is attracting growing attention. However, there remain potential issues to be solved to step forward to clinical application. The most crucial point is that we still lack ideal animal disease models for ALS. Many of the clinical trials based on experimental success unfortunately ended up with failure [140]. One possible reason is that most of the medications refer to experiments using mutant SOD1 transgenic mice. Although this ALS mouce model is indeed an excellent mimic of ALS, the dozens of higher protein expression levels are required to obtain ALS phenotypes. In this sense, recent discovery of genetic mutation in SOD1 in the paralytic dog with degenerating myelopathy casts a new light on the translation research field by providing us a new ALS model animal of natural occurrence [141]. Another theme which is prompting us to molecular targeted therapy is a concept of "prionoid hypothesis" of ALS-linked protein. In spite of the compelling evidence of *in vitro* experiments, there is no *in vivo* data, convincing us the spreading of mutant SOD1 or TDP-43. Further verification is required to justify the targeting therapy against intercellular molecules. Technically, the effective delivery of immunoglobulin to the central nervous system is another big challenge. Intrathecal route is a possible option, but its invasiveness should be well considered. In this sense, the down-sizing such as the scFv strategy, or modification to confer the better passage through the blood-brain barrier might be the next steps. Due to the various kinds of molecular engineering, intrabody strategy is expected as a new therapeutic avenue.

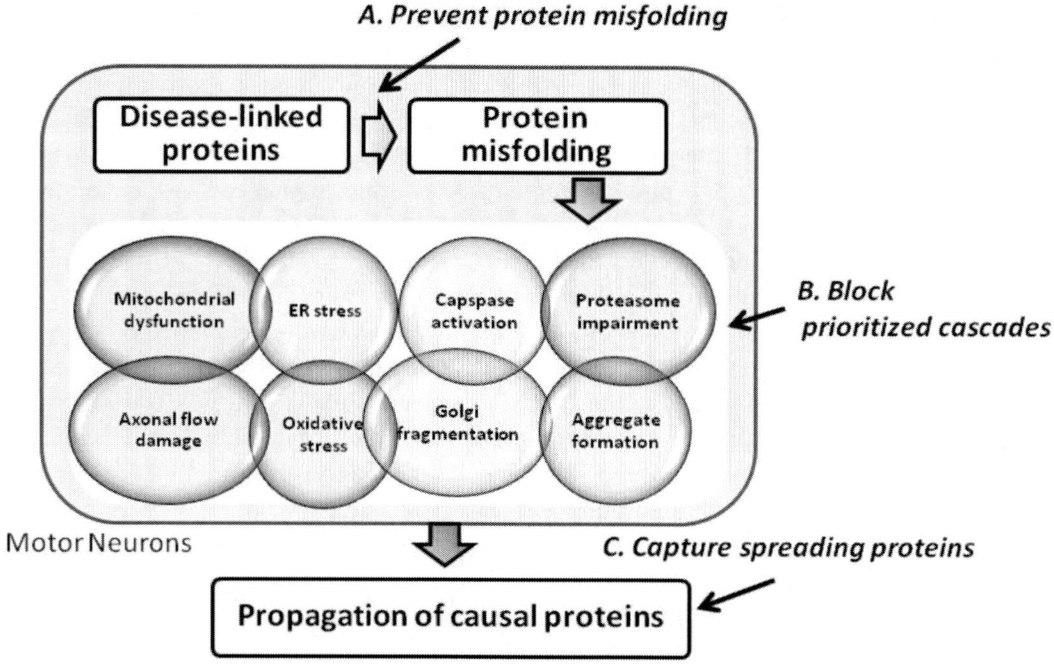

Figure 1. Schematic illustration of the cellular pathomechanisms related to ALS. Diverse pathways have been proposed to cause motor neuron death. It should be noted that many of them follow the protein misfolding of ALS-linked proteins especially in the case of mutant SOD1. Molecular targeted therapy aims to eliminate such proteins or to prevent them from conferring toxicity in the initial phase (misfolding or protein expression) as well as the later phase (propagation).

CONCLUSION

We here summarized up-to-date knowledge on the pathogenesis of ALS, especially focusing on the aberrant behavior of the causal proteins, and introduced how these proteins should be detoxified. Since antibody-antigen interaction is an ultimately specific protein-protein interaction, the further application of antibody medicine has a huge potential to expand various molecular targeted therapies.

REFERENCES

[1] Charcot JM, Joffroy A. Deux cas d'atrophie musculaire progressive avec lesions de la substance grise et des faiseaux anterolateraux de la moelle epiniere. *Archives de physiologie normale et pathologique.* 1869;2:354-67.

[2] Rothstein JD, Bristol LA, Hosler B, Brown RH, Jr., Kuncl RW. Chronic inhibition of superoxide dismutase produces apoptotic death of spinal neurons. *Proc Natl Acad Sci U S A.* 1994;91(10):4155-9. Epub 1994/05/10.

[3] Urushitani M, Shimohama S, Kihara T, Sawada H, Akaike A, Ibi M, et al. Mechanism of selective motor neuronal death after exposure of spinal cord to glutamate: involvement of glutamate-induced nitric oxide in motor neuron toxicity and nonmotor neuron protection. *Ann Neurol.* 1998;44(5):796-807. Epub 1998/11/18.

[4] Carriedo SG, Yin HZ, Sensi SL, Weiss JH. Rapid Ca2+ entry through Ca2+-permeable AMPA/Kainate channels triggers marked intracellular Ca2+ rises and consequent oxygen radical production. *J Neurosci.* 1998;18:7727-38.

[5] Michikawa M, Lim KT, McLarnon JG, Kim SU. Oxygen radical-induced neurotoxicity in spinal cord neuron cultures. *J Neurosci Res.* 1994;37(1):62-70. Epub 1994/01/01.

[6] Gendron TF, Petrucelli L. Rodent models of TDP-43 proteinopathy: investigating the mechanisms of TDP-43-mediated neurodegeneration. *J Mol Neurosci.* 2011;45(3):486-99. Epub 2011/08/04.

[7] Julien JP, Kriz J. Transgenic mouse models of amyotrophic lateral sclerosis. *Biochim Biophys Acta.* 2006;1762(11-12):1013-24. Epub 2006/05/06.

[8] Ido A, Fukuyama H, Urushitani M. Protein Misdirection Inside and Outside Motor Neurons in Amyotrophic Lateral Sclerosis (ALS): A Possible Clue for Therapeutic Strategies. *Int J Mol Sci.* 2011;12(10):6980-7003. Epub 2011/11/11.

[9] Shaw PJ. Molecular and cellular pathways of neurodegeneration in motor neurone disease. *J Neurol Neurosurg Psychiatry.* 2005;76(8):1046-57. Epub 2005/07/19.

[10] Ilieva H, Polymenidou M, Cleveland DW. Non-cell autonomous toxicity in neurodegenerative disorders: ALS and beyond. *J Cell Biol.* 2009;187(6):761-72. Epub 2009/12/03.

[11] Julien JP. Amyotrophic lateral sclerosis. unfolding the toxicity of the misfolded. *Cell.* 2001;104(4):581-91. Epub 2001/03/10.

[12] Cleveland DW, Rothstein JD. From Charcot to Lou Gehrig: deciphering selective motor neuron death in ALS. *Nature reviews Neuroscience.* 2001;2(11):806-19. Epub 2001/11/21.

[13] Lambrechts D, Robberecht W, Carmeliet P. Heterogeneity in motoneuron disease. *Trends Neurosci.* 2007;30(10):536-44. Epub 2007/09/11.

[14] Bensimon G, Lacomblez L, Meininger V. A controlled trial of riluzole in amyotrophic lateral sclerosis. ALS/Riluzole Study Group. *N Engl J Med.* 1994;330(9):585-91. Epub 1994/03/03.

[15] Lacomblez L, Bensimon G, Leigh PN, Guillet P, Powe L, Durrleman S, et al. A confirmatory dose-ranging study of riluzole in ALS. ALS/Riluzole Study Group-II. *Neurology.* 1996;47(6 Suppl 4):S242-50. Epub 1996/12/01.

[16] Wagner ML, Landis BE. Riluzole: a new agent for amyotrophic lateral sclerosis. *Ann Pharmacother.* 1997;31(6):738-44. Epub 1997/06/01.

[17] Rothstein JD, Van Kammen M, Levey AI, Martin LJ, Kuncl RW. Selective loss of glial glutamate transporter GLT-1 in amyotrophic lateral sclerosis. *Ann Neurol.* 1995;38(1):73-84. Epub 1995/07/01.

[18] Rothstein JD, Martin LJ, Kuncl RW. Decreased glutamate transport by the brain and spinal cord in amyotrophic lateral sclerosis. *N Engl J Med.* 1992;326(22):1464-8. Epub 1992/05/28.

[19] Pastula DM, Moore DH, Bedlack RS. Creatine for amyotrophic lateral sclerosis/motor neuron disease. *Cochrane database of systematic reviews.* 2010(6):CD005225. Epub 2010/06/18.

[20] Kaufmann P, Thompson JL, Levy G, Buchsbaum R, Shefner J, Krivickas LS, et al. Phase II trial of CoQ10 for ALS finds insufficient evidence to justify phase III. *Annals of neurology*. 2009;66(2):235-44. Epub 2009/09/11.

[21] Orrell RW, Lane RJ, Ross M. A systematic review of antioxidant treatment for amyotrophic lateral sclerosis/motor neuron disease. A*myotrophic lateral sclerosis : official publication of the World Federation of Neurology Research Group on Motor Neuron Diseases*. 2008;9(4):195-211. Epub 2008/07/09.

[22] Cudkowicz M, Bozik ME, Ingersoll EW, Miller R, Mitsumoto H, Shefner J, et al. The effects of dexpramipexole (KNS-760704) in individuals with amyotrophic lateral sclerosis. *Nature medicine.* 2011;17(12):1652-6. Epub 2011/11/22.

[23] Sun CN, Araoz C, Lucas G, Morgan PN, White HJ. Amyotrophic lateral sclerosis. Inclusion bodies in a case of the classic sporadic form. *Ann Clin Lab Sci.* 1975;5(1):38-44. Epub 1975/01/01.

[24] Murayama S, Ookawa Y, Mori H, Nakano I, Ihara Y, Kuzuhara S, et al. Immunocytochemical and ultrastructural study of Lewy body-like hyaline inclusions in familial amyotrophic lateral sclerosis. *Acta Neuropathol.* 1989;78(2):143-52. Epub 1989/01/01.

[25] Hirano A, Donnenfeld H, Sasaki S, Nakano I. Fine structural observations of neurofilamentous changes in amyotrophic lateral sclerosis. *J Neuropathol Exp Neurol.* 1984;43(5):461-70. Epub 1984/09/01.

[26] Takahashi K, Nakamura H, Okada E. Hereditary amyotrophic lateral sclerosis. Histochemical and electron microscopic study of hyaline inclusions in motor neurons. *Arch Neurol.* 1972;27(4):292-9. Epub 1972/10/01.

[27] Pul R, Dodel R, Stangel M. Antibody-based therapy in Alzheimer's disease. *Expert Opin Biol Ther.* 2011;11(3):343-57. Epub 2011/01/26.

[28] Watanabe M, Dykes-Hoberg M, Culotta VC, Price DL, Wong PC, Rothstein JD. Histological evidence of protein aggregation in mutant SOD1 transgenic mice and in amyotrophic lateral sclerosis neural tissues. *Neurobiol Dis.* 2001;8(6):933-41. Epub 2001/12/14.

[29] Urushitani M, Kurisu J, Tateno M, Hatakeyama S, Nakayama K, Kato S, et al. CHIP promotes proteasomal degradation of familial ALS-linked mutant SOD1 by ubiquitinating Hsp/Hsc70. *J Neurochem.* 2004;90(1):231-44. Epub 2004/06/17.

[30] Kabuta T, Suzuki Y, Wada K. Degradation of amyotrophic lateral sclerosis-linked mutant Cu,Zn-superoxide dismutase proteins by macroautophagy and the proteasome. *J Biol Chem*. 2006;281(41):30524-33. Epub 2006/08/22.

[31] Hetz C, Thielen P, Matus S, Nassif M, Court F, Kiffin R, et al. XBP-1 deficiency in the nervous system protects against amyotrophic lateral sclerosis by increasing autophagy. *Genes Dev*. 2009;23(19):2294-306. Epub 2009/09/19.

[32] Urushitani M, Kurisu J, Tsukita K, Takahashi R. Proteasomal inhibition by misfolded mutant superoxide dismutase 1 induces selective motor neuron death in familial amyotrophic lateral sclerosis. *J Neurochem*. 2002;83(5):1030-42. Epub 2002/11/20.

[33] Waxman EA, Giasson BI. Molecular mechanisms of alpha-synuclein neurodegeneration. *Biochimica et biophysica acta*. 2009;1792(7):616-24. Epub 2008/10/29.

[34] Schenk D, Barbour R, Dunn W, Gordon G, Grajeda H, Guido T, et al. Immunization with amyloid-beta attenuates Alzheimer-disease-like pathology in the PDAPP mouse. *Nature*. 1999;400(6740):173-7.

[35] McLaurin J, Cecal R, Kierstead ME, Tian X, Phinney AL, Manea M, et al. Therapeutically effective antibodies against amyloid-beta peptide target amyloid-beta residues 4-10 and inhibit cytotoxicity and fibrillogenesis. *Nat Med*. 2002;8(11):1263-9.

[36] Masliah E, Rockenstein E, Adame A, Alford M, Crews L, Hashimoto M, et al. Effects of alpha-Synuclein Immunization in a Mouse Model of Parkinson's Disease. *Neuron*. 2005;46(6):857-68.

[37] Urushitani M, Ezzi SA, Julien JP. Therapeutic effects of immunization with mutant superoxide dismutase in mice models of amyotrophic lateral sclerosis. *Proc Natl Acad Sci U S A*. 2007;104(7):2495-500. Epub 2007/02/06.

[38] Takeuchi S, Fujiwara N, Ido A, Oono M, Takeuchi Y, Tateno M, et al. Induction of protective immunity by vaccination with wild-type apo superoxide dismutase 1 in mutant SOD1 transgenic mice. *J Neuropathol Exp Neurol*. 2010;69(10):1044-56. Epub 2010/09/15.

[39] Rosen DR, Siddique T, Patterson D, Figlewicz DA, Sapp P, Hentati A, et al. Mutations in Cu/Zn superoxide dismutase gene are associated with familial amyotrophic lateral sclerosis. *Nature*. 1993;362:59-62.

[40] Reaume AG, Elliott JL, Hoffman EK, Kowall NW, Ferrante RJ, Siwek DF, et al. Motor neurons in Cu/Zn superoxide dismutase-deficient mice develop normally but exhibit enhanced cell death after axonal injury. *Nat Genet*. 1996;13(Ref #485 of 1261 in SOD.REF):43-7.

[41] Wang J, Xu G, Gonzales V, Coonfield M, Fromholt D, Copeland NG, et al. Fibrillar inclusions and motor neuron degeneration in transgenic mice expressing superoxide dismutase 1 with a disrupted copper-binding site. *Neurobiol Dis*. 2002;10(2):128-38. Epub 2002/07/20.

[42] Tiwari A, Hayward LJ. Familial amyotrophic lateral sclerosis mutants of copper/zinc superoxide dismutase are susceptible to disulfide reduction. *J Biol Chem*. 2003;278(8):5984-92. Epub 2002/11/30.

[43] Furukawa Y, Kaneko K, Yamanaka K, Nukina N. Mutation-dependent polymorphism of Cu,Zn-superoxide dismutase aggregates in the familial form of amyotrophic lateral sclerosis. *J Biol Chem*. 2010;285(29):22221-31. Epub 2010/04/21.

[44] Valentine JS, Hart PJ. Misfolded CuZnSOD and amyotrophic lateral sclerosis. *Proc Natl Acad Sci U S A*. 2003;100(7):3617-22. Epub 2003/03/26.

[45] Israelson A, Arbel N, Da Cruz S, Ilieva H, Yamanaka K, Shoshan-Barmatz V, et al. Misfolded mutant SOD1 directly inhibits VDAC1 conductance in a mouse model of inherited ALS. *Neuron*. 2010;67(4):575-87. Epub 2010/08/28.

[46] Kikuchi H, Almer G, Yamashita S, Guegan C, Nagai M, Xu Z, et al. Spinal cord endoplasmic reticulum stress associated with a microsomal accumulation of mutant superoxide dismutase-1 in an ALS model. *Proc Natl Acad Sci U S A*. 2006;103(15):6025-30. Epub 2006/04/06.

[47] Nishitoh H, Kadowaki H, Nagai A, Maruyama T, Yokota T, Fukutomi H, et al. ALS-linked mutant SOD1 induces ER stress- and ASK1-dependent motor neuron death by targeting Derlin-1. *Genes Dev*. 2008;22(11):1451-64. Epub 2008/06/04.

[48] Urushitani M, Sik A, Sakurai T, Nukina N, Takahashi R, Julien JP. Chromogranin-mediated secretion of mutant superoxide dismutase proteins linked to amyotrophic lateral sclerosis. *Nat Neurosci*. 2006;9(1):108-18. Epub 2005/12/22.

[49] Sargsyan SA, Blackburn DJ, Barber SC, Grosskreutz J, De Vos KJ, Monk PN, et al. A comparison of *in vitro* properties of resting SOD1 transgenic microglia reveals evidence of reduced neuroprotective function. *BMC neuroscience*. 2011;12:91. Epub 2011/09/29.

[50] Vargas MR, Pehar M, Diaz-Amarilla PJ, Beckman JS, Barbeito L. Transcriptional profile of primary astrocytes expressing ALS-linked mutant SOD1. *J Neurosci Res*. 2008;86(16):3515-25. Epub 2008/08/07.

[51] Di Giorgio FP, Boulting GL, Bobrowicz S, Eggan KC. Human embryonic stem cell-derived motor neurons are sensitive to the toxic effect of glial cells carrying an ALS-causing mutation. *Cell stem cell*. 2008;3(6):637-48. Epub 2008/12/02.

[52] Lino MM, Schneider C, Caroni P. Accumulation of SOD1 mutants in postnatal motoneurons does not cause motoneuron pathology or motoneuron disease. *J Neurosci*. 2002;22(12):4825-32.

[53] Gong YH, Parsadanian AS, Andreeva A, Snider WD, Elliott JL. Restricted expression of G86R Cu/Zn superoxide dismutase in astrocytes results in astrocytosis but does not cause motoneuron degeneration. *J Neurosci*. 2000;20(Ref #247 of 1261 in SOD.REF):660-5.

[54] Beers DR, Henkel JS, Xiao Q, Zhao W, Wang J, Yen AA, et al. Wild-type microglia extend survival in PU.1 knockout mice with familial amyotrophic lateral sclerosis. *Proc Natl Acad Sci U S A*. 2006;103(43):16021-6.

[55] Pramatarova A, Laganiere J, Roussel J, Brisebois K, Rouleau GA. Neuron-specific expression of mutant superoxide dismutase 1 in transgenic mice does not lead to motor impairment. *J Neurosci*. 2001;21(10):3369-74. Epub 2001/05/23.

[56] Clement AM, Nguyen MD, Roberts EA, Garcia ML, Boillee S, Rule M, et al. Wild-type nonneuronal cells extend survival of SOD1 mutant motor neurons in ALS mice. *Science*. 2003;302(5642):113-7. Epub 2003/10/04.

[57] Boillee S, Yamanaka K, Lobsiger CS, Copeland NG, Jenkins NA, Kassiotis G, et al. Onset and progression in inherited ALS determined by motor neurons and microglia. *Science*. 2006;312(5778):1389-92. Epub 2006/06/03.

[58] Yamanaka K, Chun SJ, Boillee S, Fujimori-Tonou N, Yamashita H, Gutmann DH, et al. Astrocytes as determinants of disease progression in inherited amyotrophic lateral sclerosis. *Nat Neurosci*. 2008;11(3):251-3.

[59] Nagai M, Re DB, Nagata T, Chalazonitis A, Jessell TM, Wichterle H, et al. Astrocytes expressing ALS-linked mutated SOD1 release factors selectively toxic to motor neurons. *Nat Neurosci*. 2007;10(5):615-22. Epub 2007/04/17.

[60] Papadeas ST, Kraig SE, O'Banion C, Lepore AC, Maragakis NJ. Astrocytes carrying the superoxide dismutase 1 (SOD1G93A) mutation induce wild-type motor neuron

degeneration *in vivo*. *Proc Natl Acad Sci U S A*. 2011;108(43):17803-8. Epub 2011/10/05.

[61] Wang L, Sharma K, Deng HX, Siddique T, Grisotti G, Liu E, et al. Restricted expression of mutant SOD1 in spinal motor neurons and interneurons induces motor neuron pathology. *Neurobiol Dis*. 2008;29(3):400-8. Epub 2007/12/07.

[62] Wang L, Gutmann DH, Roos RP. Astrocyte loss of mutant SOD1 delays ALS disease onset and progression in G85R transgenic mice. *Hum Mol Genet*. 2011;20(2):286-93. Epub 2010/10/22.

[63] Appel SH, Beers DR, Henkel JS. T cell-microglial dialogue in Parkinson's disease and amyotrophic lateral sclerosis: are we listening? *Trends Immunol*. 2010;31(1):7-17. Epub 2009/11/03.

[64] Kiaei M, Kipiani K, Calingasan NY, Wille E, Chen J, Heissig B, et al. Matrix metalloproteinase-9 regulates TNF-alpha and FasL expression in neuronal, glial cells and its absence extends life in a transgenic mouse model of amyotrophic lateral sclerosis. *Exp Neurol*. 2007;205(1):74-81. Epub 2007/03/17.

[65] Gros-Louis F, Andersen PM, Dupre N, Urushitani M, Dion P, Souchon F, et al. Chromogranin B P413L variant as risk factor and modifier of disease onset for amyotrophic lateral sclerosis. *Proc Natl Acad Sci U S A*. 2009;106(51):21777-82. Epub 2009/12/17.

[66] Zhao W, Beers DR, Henkel JS, Zhang W, Urushitani M, Julien JP, et al. Extracellular mutant SOD1 induces microglial-mediated motoneuron injury. *Glia*. 2010;58(2):231-43. Epub 2009/08/13.

[67] Schrott-Fischer A, Bitsche M, Humpel C, Walcher C, Maier H, Jellinger K, et al. Chromogranin peptides in amyotrophic lateral sclerosis. *Regul Pept*. 2009;152(1-3):13-21. Epub 2008/08/30.

[68] Zetterstrom P, Andersen PM, Brannstrom T, Marklund SL. Misfolded superoxide dismutase-1 in CSF from amyotrophic lateral sclerosis patients. *J Neurochem*. 2011;117(1):91-9. Epub 2011/01/14.

[69] Ezzi SA, Urushitani M, Julien JP. Wild-type superoxide dismutase acquires binding and toxic properties of ALS-linked mutant forms through oxidation. *J Neurochem*. 2007;102(1):170-8. Epub 2007/03/31.

[70] Munch C, O'Brien J, Bertolotti A. Prion-like propagation of mutant superoxide dismutase-1 misfolding in neuronal cells. *Proc Natl Acad Sci U S A*. 2011;108(9):3548-53. Epub 2011/02/16.

[71] Chia R, Tattum MH, Jones S, Collinge J, Fisher EM, Jackson GS. Superoxide dismutase 1 and tgSOD1 mouse spinal cord seed fibrils, suggesting a propagative cell death mechanism in amyotrophic lateral sclerosis. *PloS one*. 2010;5(5):e10627. Epub 2010/05/26.

[72] Grad LI, Guest WC, Yanai A, Pokrishevsky E, O'Neill MA, Gibbs E, et al. Intermolecular transmission of superoxide dismutase 1 misfolding in living cells. *Proc Natl Acad Sci U S A*. 2011;108(39):16398-403. Epub 2011/09/21.

[73] Gros-Louis F, Soucy G, Lariviere R, Julien JP. Intracerebroventricular infusion of monoclonal antibody or its derived Fab fragment against misfolded forms of SOD1 mutant delays mortality in a mouse model of ALS. *J Neurochem*. 2010;113(5):1188-99. Epub 2010/03/30.

[74] Elam JS, Taylor AB, Strange R, Antonyuk S, Doucette PA, Rodriguez JA, et al. Amyloid-like filaments and water-filled nanotubes formed by SOD1 mutant proteins linked to familial ALS. *Nat Struct Biol.* 2003;10(6):461-7. Epub 2003/05/20.

[75] Shibata N, Hirano A, Kobayashi M, Dal Canto MC, Gurney ME, Komori T, et al. Presence of Cu/Zn superoxide dismutase (SOD) immunoreactivity in neuronal hyaline inclusions in spinal cords from mice carrying a transgene for Gly93Ala mutant human Cu/Zn SOD. *Acta Neuropathol.* 1998;95(2):136-42. Epub 1998/03/14.

[76] Gruzman A, Wood WL, Alpert E, Prasad MD, Miller RG, Rothstein JD, et al. Common molecular signature in SOD1 for both sporadic and familial amyotrophic lateral sclerosis. *Proc Natl Acad Sci U S A.* 2007;104(30):12524-9. Epub 2007/07/20.

[77] Bosco DA, Morfini G, Karabacak NM, Song Y, Gros-Louis F, Pasinelli P, et al. Wild-type and mutant SOD1 share an aberrant conformation and a common pathogenic pathway in ALS. *Nat Neurosci.* 2010;13(11):1396-403. Epub 2010/10/19.

[78] Haidet-Phillips AM, Hester ME, Miranda CJ, Meyer K, Braun L, Frakes A, et al. Astrocytes from familial and sporadic ALS patients are toxic to motor neurons. *Nat Biotechnol.* 2011;29(9):824-8. Epub 2011/08/13.

[79] Brotherton TE, Li Y, Cooper D, Gearing M, Julien JP, Rothstein JD, et al. Localization of a toxic form of superoxide dismutase 1 protein to pathologically affected tissues in familial ALS. *Proc Natl Acad Sci U S A.* 2012. Epub 2012/03/21.

[80] Liu HN, Sanelli T, Horne P, Pioro EP, Strong MJ, Rogaeva E, et al. Lack of evidence of monomer/misfolded superoxide dismutase-1 in sporadic amyotrophic lateral sclerosis. *Ann Neurol.* 2009;66(1):75-80. Epub 2009/08/12.

[81] Arai T, Hasegawa M, Akiyama H, Ikeda K, Nonaka T, Mori H, et al. TDP-43 is a component of ubiquitin-positive tau-negative inclusions in frontotemporal lobar degeneration and amyotrophic lateral sclerosis. *Biochem Biophys Res Commun.* 2006;351(3):602-11. Epub 2006/11/07.

[82] Neumann M, Sampathu DM, Kwong LK, Truax AC, Micsenyi MC, Chou TT, et al. Ubiquitinated TDP-43 in frontotemporal lobar degeneration and amyotrophic lateral sclerosis. *Science.* 2006;314(5796):130-3. Epub 2006/10/07.

[83] Davidson Y, Kelley T, Mackenzie IR, Pickering-Brown S, Du Plessis D, Neary D, et al. Ubiquitinated pathological lesions in frontotemporal lobar degeneration contain the TAR DNA-binding protein, TDP-43. *Acta Neuropathol.* 2007;113(5):521-33. Epub 2007/01/16.

[84] Cairns NJ, Neumann M, Bigio EH, Holm IE, Troost D, Hatanpaa KJ, et al. TDP-43 in familial and sporadic frontotemporal lobar degeneration with ubiquitin inclusions. *Am J Pathol.* 2007;171(1):227-40. Epub 2007/06/27.

[85] Gitcho MA, Baloh RH, Chakraverty S, Mayo K, Norton JB, Levitch D, et al. TDP-43 A315T mutation in familial motor neuron disease. *Ann Neurol.* 2008;63(4):535-8. Epub 2008/02/22.

[86] Yokoseki A, Shiga A, Tan CF, Tagawa A, Kaneko H, Koyama A, et al. TDP-43 mutation in familial amyotrophic lateral sclerosis. *Ann Neurol.* 2008;63(4):538-42. Epub 2008/04/29.

[87] Corrado L, Ratti A, Gellera C, Buratti E, Castellotti B, Carlomagno Y, et al. High frequency of TARDBP gene mutations in Italian patients with amyotrophic lateral sclerosis. *Hum Mutat.* 2009;30(4):688-94. Epub 2009/02/19.

[88] Van Deerlin VM, Leverenz JB, Bekris LM, Bird TD, Yuan W, Elman LB, et al. TARDBP mutations in amyotrophic lateral sclerosis with TDP-43 neuropathology: a genetic and histopathological analysis. *Lancet Neurol.* 2008;7(5):409-16. Epub 2008/04/09.

[89] Kabashi E, Valdmanis PN, Dion P, Spiegelman D, McConkey BJ, Vande Velde C, et al. TARDBP mutations in individuals with sporadic and familial amyotrophic lateral sclerosis. *Nat Genet*. 2008;40(5):572-4. Epub 2008/04/01.

[90] Sreedharan J, Blair IP, Tripathi VB, Hu X, Vance C, Rogelj B, et al. TDP-43 mutations in familial and sporadic amyotrophic lateral sclerosis. *Science*. 2008;319(5870):1668-72. Epub 2008/03/01.

[91] Wu LS, Cheng WC, Hou SC, Yan YT, Jiang ST, Shen CK. TDP-43, a neuro-pathosignature factor, is essential for early mouse embryogenesis. *Genesis*. 2010;48(1):56-62. Epub 2009/12/17.

[92] Chiang PM, Ling J, Jeong YH, Price DL, Aja SM, Wong PC. Deletion of TDP-43 down-regulates Tbc1d1, a gene linked to obesity, and alters body fat metabolism. *Proc Natl Acad Sci U S A*. 2010;107(37):16320-4. Epub 2010/07/28.

[93] Caccamo A, Majumder S, Oddo S. Cognitive decline typical of frontotemporal lobar degeneration in transgenic mice expressing the 25-kDa C-terminal fragment of TDP-43. *Am J Pathol.* 2012;180(1):293-302. Epub 2011/11/10.

[94] Swarup V, Phaneuf D, Bareil C, Robertson J, Rouleau GA, Kriz J, et al. Pathological hallmarks of amyotrophic lateral sclerosis/frontotemporal lobar degeneration in transgenic mice produced with TDP-43 genomic fragments. *Brain*. 2011;134(Pt 9):2610-26. Epub 2011/07/15.

[95] Igaz LM, Kwong LK, Lee EB, Chen-Plotkin A, Swanson E, Unger T, et al. Dysregulation of the ALS-associated gene TDP-43 leads to neuronal death and degeneration in mice. *J Clin Invest.* 2011;121(2):726-38. Epub 2011/01/06.

[96] Xu YF, Gendron TF, Zhang YJ, Lin WL, D'Alton S, Sheng H, et al. Wild-type human TDP-43 expression causes TDP-43 phosphorylation, mitochondrial aggregation, motor deficits, and early mortality in transgenic mice. *J Neurosci.* 2010;30(32):10851-9. Epub 2010/08/13.

[97] Stallings NR, Puttaparthi K, Luther CM, Burns DK, Elliott JL. Progressive motor weakness in transgenic mice expressing human TDP-43. *Neurobiol Dis.* 2010;40(2):404-14. Epub 2010/07/14.

[98] Shan X, Chiang PM, Price DL, Wong PC. Altered distributions of Gemini of coiled bodies and mitochondria in motor neurons of TDP-43 transgenic mice. *Proc Natl Acad Sci U S A*. 2010;107(37):16325-30. Epub 2010/08/26.

[99] Wegorzewska I, Bell S, Cairns NJ, Miller TM, Baloh RH. TDP-43 mutant transgenic mice develop features of ALS and frontotemporal lobar degeneration. *Proc Natl Acad Sci U S A.* 2009;106(44):18809-14. Epub 2009/10/17.

[100] Wils H, Kleinberger G, Janssens J, Pereson S, Joris G, Cuijt I, et al. TDP-43 transgenic mice develop spastic paralysis and neuronal inclusions characteristic of ALS and frontotemporal lobar degeneration. *Proc Natl Acad Sci U S A.* 2010;107(8):3858-63. Epub 2010/02/06.

[101] Swarup V, Phaneuf D, Dupre N, Petri S, Strong M, Kriz J, et al. Deregulation of TDP-43 in amyotrophic lateral sclerosis triggers nuclear factor kappaB-mediated pathogenic pathways. *J Exp Med.* 2011;208(12):2429-47. Epub 2011/11/16.

[102] Zhang YJ, Xu YF, Dickey CA, Buratti E, Baralle F, Bailey R, et al. Progranulin mediates caspase-dependent cleavage of TAR DNA binding protein-43. *J Neurosci.* 2007;27(39):10530-4. Epub 2007/09/28.

[103] Ling SC, Albuquerque CP, Han JS, Lagier-Tourenne C, Tokunaga S, Zhou H, et al. ALS-associated mutations in TDP-43 increase its stability and promote TDP-43 complexes with FUS/TLS. *Proc Natl Acad Sci U S A.* 2010;107(30):13318-23. Epub 2010/07/14.

[104] Ayala YM, Misteli T, Baralle FE. TDP-43 regulates retinoblastoma protein phosphorylation through the repression of cyclin-dependent kinase 6 expression. *Proc Natl Acad Sci U S A.* 2008;105(10):3785-9. Epub 2008/02/29.

[105] Fiesel FC, Voigt A, Weber SS, Van den Haute C, Waldenmaier A, Gorner K, et al. Knockdown of transactive response DNA-binding protein (TDP-43) downregulates histone deacetylase 6. *EMBO J.* 2010;29(1):209-21. Epub 2009/11/17.

[106] Iguchi Y, Katsuno M, Niwa J, Yamada S, Sone J, Waza M, et al. TDP-43 depletion induces neuronal cell damage through dysregulation of Rho family GTPases. *J Biol Chem.* 2009;284(33):22059-66. Epub 2009/06/19.

[107] Buratti E, De Conti L, Stuani C, Romano M, Baralle M, Baralle F. Nuclear factor TDP-43 can affect selected microRNA levels. *The FEBS journal.* 2010;277(10):2268-81. Epub 2010/04/29.

[108] Xiao S, Sanelli T, Dib S, Sheps D, Findlater J, Bilbao J, et al. RNA targets of TDP-43 identified by UV-CLIP are deregulated in ALS. *Mol Cell Neurosci.* 2011;47(3):167-80. Epub 2011/03/23.

[109] Polymenidou M, Lagier-Tourenne C, Hutt KR, Huelga SC, Moran J, Liang TY, et al. Long pre-mRNA depletion and RNA missplicing contribute to neuronal vulnerability from loss of TDP-43. *Nat Neurosci.* 2011;14(4):459-68. Epub 2011/03/02.

[110] Tollervey JR, Curk T, Rogelj B, Briese M, Cereda M, Kayikci M, et al. Characterizing the RNA targets and position-dependent splicing regulation by TDP-43. *Nat Neurosci.* 2011;14(4):452-8. Epub 2011/03/02.

[111] Huang C, Zhou H, Tong J, Chen H, Liu YJ, Wang D, et al. FUS transgenic rats develop the phenotypes of amyotrophic lateral sclerosis and frontotemporal lobar degeneration. *PLoS genetics.* 2011;7(3):e1002011. Epub 2011/03/17.

[112] Rezaie T, Child A, Hitchings R, Brice G, Miller L, Coca-Prados M, et al. Adult-onset primary open-angle glaucoma caused by mutations in optineurin. *Science.* 2002;295(5557):1077-9. Epub 2002/02/09.

[113] Maruyama H, Morino H, Ito H, Izumi Y, Kato H, Watanabe Y, et al. Mutations of optineurin in amyotrophic lateral sclerosis. *Nature.* 2010;465(7295):223-6. Epub 2010/04/30.

[114] Solski JA, Williams KL, Yang S, Nicholson GA, Blair IP. Mutation analysis of the optineurin gene in familial amyotrophic lateral sclerosis. *Neurobiol Aging.* 2012;33(1):210 e9-10. Epub 2011/10/22.

[115] Millecamps S, Boillee S, Chabrol E, Camu W, Cazeneuve C, Salachas F, et al. Screening of OPTN in French familial amyotrophic lateral sclerosis. *Neurobiol Aging.* 2011;32(3):557 e11-3. Epub 2011/01/12.

[116] Weidberg H, Elazar Z. TBK1 mediates crosstalk between the innate immune response and autophagy. *Science signaling.* 2011;4(187):pe39. Epub 2011/08/27.

[117] Ralph GS, Radcliffe PA, Day DM, Carthy JM, Leroux MA, Lee DC, et al. Silencing mutant SOD1 using RNAi protects against neurodegeneration and extends survival in an ALS model. *Nat Med.* 2005;11(4):429-33. Epub 2005/03/16.

[118] Raoul C, Abbas-Terki T, Bensadoun JC, Guillot S, Haase G, Szulc J, et al. Lentiviral-mediated silencing of SOD1 through RNA interference retards disease onset and progression in a mouse model of ALS. *Nat Med.* 2005;11(4):423-8. Epub 2005/03/16.

[119] Smith RA, Miller TM, Yamanaka K, Monia BP, Condon TP, Hung G, et al. Antisense oligonucleotide therapy for neurodegenerative disease. *J Clin Invest.* 2006;116(8):2290-6. Epub 2006/08/01.

[120] Johnston JA, Dalton MJ, Gurney ME, Kopito RR. Formation of high molecular weight complexes of mutant Cu, Zn-superoxide dismutase in a mouse model for familial amyotrophic lateral sclerosis. *Proc Natl Acad Sci U S A.* 2000;97(23):12571-6. Epub 2000/10/26.

[121] Niwa J, Ishigaki S, Hishikawa N, Yamamoto M, Doyu M, Murata S, et al. Dorfin ubiquitylates mutant SOD1 and prevents mutant SOD1-mediated neurotoxicity. *J Biol Chem.* 2002;277(39):36793-8. Epub 2002/07/30.

[122] Miyazaki K, Fujita T, Ozaki T, Kato C, Kurose Y, Sakamoto M, et al. NEDL1, a novel ubiquitin-protein isopeptide ligase for dishevelled-1, targets mutant superoxide dismutase-1. *J Biol Chem.* 2004;279(12):11327-35. Epub 2003/12/20.

[123] Sone J, Niwa J, Kawai K, Ishigaki S, Yamada S, Adachi H, et al. Dorfin ameliorates phenotypes in a transgenic mouse model of amyotrophic lateral sclerosis. *J Neurosci Res.* 2010;88(1):123-35. Epub 2009/07/18.

[124] Zhang L, Haraguchi S, Koda T, Hashimoto K, Nakagawara A. Muscle atrophy and motor neuron degeneration in human NEDL1 transgenic mice. *Journal of biomedicine & biotechnology.* 2011;2011:831092. Epub 2010/10/27.

[125] Urushitani M, Sato T, Bamba H, Hisa Y, Tooyama I. Synergistic effect between proteasome and autophagosome in the clearance of polyubiquitinated TDP-43. *J Neurosci Res.* 2010;88(4):784-97. Epub 2009/10/03.

[126] Bhattacharya A, Bokov A, Muller FL, Jernigan AL, Maslin K, Diaz V, et al. Dietary restriction but not rapamycin extends disease onset and survival of the H46R/H48Q mouse model of ALS. *Neurobiol Aging.* 2011. Epub 2011/07/19.

[127] Feldman ME, Apsel B, Uotila A, Loewith R, Knight ZA, Ruggero D, et al. Active-site inhibitors of mTOR target rapamycin-resistant outputs of mTORC1 and mTORC2. *PLoS biology.* 2009;7(2):e38. Epub 2009/02/13.

[128] Thoreen CC, Kang SA, Chang JW, Liu Q, Zhang J, Gao Y, et al. An ATP-competitive mammalian target of rapamycin inhibitor reveals rapamycin-resistant functions of mTORC1. *J Biol Chem.* 2009;284(12):8023-32. Epub 2009/01/20.

[129] Furukawa Y, Fu R, Deng HX, Siddique T, O'Halloran TV. Disulfide cross-linked protein represents a significant fraction of ALS-associated Cu, Zn-superoxide dismutase aggregates in spinal cords of model mice. *Proc Natl Acad Sci U S A.* 2006;103(18):7148-53. Epub 2006/04/26.

[130] Fujiwara N, Nakano M, Kato S, Yoshihara D, Ookawara T, Eguchi H, et al. Oxidative modification to cysteine sulfonic acid of Cys111 in human copper-zinc superoxide dismutase. *J Biol Chem.* 2007;282(49):35933-44. Epub 2007/10/05.

[131] Watanabe S, Nagano S, Duce J, Kiaei M, Li QX, Tucker SM, et al. Increased affinity for copper mediated by cysteine 111 in forms of mutant superoxide dismutase 1 linked

to amyotrophic lateral sclerosis. *Free Radic Biol Med.* 2007;42(10):1534-42. Epub 2007/04/24.

[132] Hernandez S, Casanovas A, Piedrafita L, Tarabal O, Esquerda JE. Neurotoxic species of misfolded SOD1G93A recognized by antibodies against the P2X4 subunit of the ATP receptor accumulate in damaged neurons of transgenic animal models of amyotrophic lateral sclerosis. *J Neuropathol Exp Neurol.* 2010;69(2):176-87. Epub 2010/01/20.

[133] Teilum K, Smith MH, Schulz E, Christensen LC, Solomentsev G, Oliveberg M, et al. Transient structural distortion of metal-free Cu/Zn superoxide dismutase triggers aberrant oligomerization. *Proc Natl Acad Sci U S A.* 2009;106(43):18273-8. Epub 2009/10/16.

[134] Zhang W, Benmohamed R, Arvanites AC, Morimoto RI, Ferrante RJ, Kirsch DR, et al. Cyclohexane 1,3-diones and their inhibition of mutant SOD1-dependent protein aggregation and toxicity in PC12 cells. *Bioorg Med Chem.* 2012;20(2):1029-45. Epub 2011/12/23.

[135] Murakami G, Inoue H, Tsukita K, Asai Y, Amagai Y, Aiba K, et al. Chemical library screening identifies a small molecule that downregulates SOD1 transcription for drugs to treat amyotrophic lateral sclerosis. *Journal of biomolecular screening.* 2011;16(4):405-14. Epub 2011/03/03.

[136] Furukawa Y, Kaneko K, Watanabe S, Yamanaka K, Nukina N. A seeding reaction recapitulates intracellular formation of Sarkosyl-insoluble transactivation response element (TAR) DNA-binding protein-43 inclusions. *J Biol Chem.* 2011;286(21):18664-72. Epub 2011/04/02.

[137] Cohen TJ, Hwang AW, Unger T, Trojanowski JQ, Lee VM. Redox signalling directly regulates TDP-43 via cysteine oxidation and disulphide cross-linking. *EMBO J.* 2012;31(5):1241-52. Epub 2011/12/24.

[138] Emadi S, Kasturirangan S, Wang MS, Schulz P, Sierks MR. Detecting morphologically distinct oligomeric forms of alpha-synuclein. *J Biol Chem.* 2009;284(17):11048-58. Epub 2009/01/15.

[139] Wang YJ, Gao CY, Yang M, Liu XH, Sun Y, Pollard A, et al. Intramuscular delivery of a single chain antibody gene prevents brain Abeta deposition and cognitive impairment in a mouse model of Alzheimer's disease. *Brain Behav Immun.* 2010;24(8):1281-93. Epub 2010/07/03.

[140] Gordon PH, Meininger V. How can we improve clinical trials in amyotrophic lateral sclerosis? *Nature reviews Neurology.* 2011;7(11):650-4. Epub 2011/09/29.

[141] Awano T, Johnson GS, Wade CM, Katz ML, Johnson GC, Taylor JF, et al. Genome-wide association analysis reveals a SOD1 mutation in canine degenerative myelopathy that resembles amyotrophic lateral sclerosis. *Proc Natl Acad Sci U S A.* 2009;106(8):2794-9. Epub 2009/02/04.

In: Amyotrophic Lateral Sclerosis
Editors: Katashi Segawa and Ryota Ijichi ISBN: 978-1-62257-679-1

Chapter 4

Amyotrophic Lateral Sclerosis: Exploring the Impact of Decreased Speech Intelligibility on Marital Communication

Karin Joubert
University of the Witwatersrand, Johannesburg, South Africa

ABSTRACT

Background: The physical and communication disabilities resulting from the onset of amyotrophic lateral sclerosis (ALS) impinge on individuals' ability to remain functionally independent. This decrease in independence inevitably leads to continuously changing roles and responsibilities within the marital relationship. One of the most constructive ways in dealing with the emotions elicited by these changes is communication.

Method: This correlational study aimed to explore the relationship between the deteriorating speech of persons with ALS and the couple's perception of marital communication. Fourteen couples participated in this study. Data were collected at three-monthly intervals over a 12-month period through the administration of objective and subjective measures.

Results: The results of the study confirmed the inevitable decline in speech intelligibility across the disease progression. However, despite this decline, the relationship between the deteriorating speech and the couples' perception of marital communication was not statistically significant.

Conclusions: The assumption that communication between couples will invariably deteriorate as a result of gradually decreasing speech intelligibility is not necessarily valid. This highlights the vital importance of effective marital communication. The use of effective augmentative and alternative communication strategies has been proven to preserve the ability to develop and maintain intimate, rewarding relationships despite the presence of profound physical disabilities.

Keywords: Speech intelligibility, marital communication, augmentative and alternative communication, spouses

Impact of ALS on the Individual

Individuals diagnosed with a gradual onset, progressive disease such as amyotrophic lateral sclerosis (ALS) require constant, protracted periods of adapting to the decline in physical and communication abilities (Lasker and Bedrosian, 2000; Mathy, Yorkston and Gutmann, 2000). Adapting can be defined as "altering life and self to accommodate to bodily losses and limits and resolving the lost unity between body and self" (Charmaz, 1995, p. 657). This adaptation process comprises three major stages that seldom only occur once, but rather repeatedly, as individuals continually experience new losses. The first stage includes the experiencing and defining of impairment. The second stage, making bodily assessment, subsequently requires identity trade-offs as individuals weigh their losses and gains, resulting in revised identity goals. The last stage involves relinquishing control over the illness and flowing with the experience of it (Charmaz, 1995, p. 657). Further to this, the International Classification of Functioning, Disability and Health (ICF) provide a framework for describing the impact of ALS on the levels of activity, participation, environmental and personal factors (World Health Organization [WHO], 2001). Both the adaptation to illness model and the ICF is particularly pertinent to persons with ALS (PALS) who experience increasing physical and communication impairment.

Physical Abilities

PALS will invariably experience increasing physical impairment as a result of relentless progressive muscular weakness. The decline in muscular function may negatively impact on mobility (e.g. walking, dressing, driving), digestive function and structure (e.g. eating as a result of dysphagia) and respiration (e.g. breathing). Performing these functions will become progressively more difficult until ultimately dependence in most of these areas is inevitable (Lasker and Bedrosian, 2000). This will require a constant process of adapting to one loss of physical function before another presents itself (Mathy et al., 2000; McLeod and Clarke, 2007).

Communication Abilities

One of the most profound changes that PALS may experience is the loss of voice and speech function (Fox and Sohlberg, 2000; Lasker and Bedrosian, 2000; Light, Arnold, and Clark, 2003). Speech, one of the principal forms of communication, is used in every facet of our lives. The rapid decline of speech function as a result of dysarthria is common as between 75% and 80% of PALS will reach a point where intelligible verbal communication is no longer possible (Ball, Beukelman and Pattee, 2004; Kuhnlein et al. 2008; Leigh et al., 2003). Dysarthria, a motor speech disorder that results from damage to the peripheral or central nervous system, is characterized by the imprecision of the movement of the speech musculature (Darley, Aronson and Brown, 1969). This imprecision can be the result of impaired muscle tone affecting the range and power of the voice, breathing, oral movements as well as the in-coordination of the speech musculature (Duffy, 1995). The speech sub-scale of the ALS Severity Scale (ALSSS) developed by Hillel et al. (1989) allows for accurate assessment of the functional impairment that PALS present with in the area of speech, with speech intelligibility specifically used as the indicator of functional impairment across the disease progression. This was used by Yorkston, Miller and Strand (1995) to further describe the typical progression of dysarthria in PALS. In the early stage (Stage 1), no obvious deficits are noticeable in an individuals' speech, but as the disease progresses, speech intelligibility becomes more compromised until when at the 5th and final stage, individuals lose all speech function.

Speech intelligibility is defined as the accuracy with which a spoken utterance is conveyed by the speaker and understood by the listener (Yorkston et al., 1999; Yunusova et al., 2005). Sentence intelligibility measures, such as the Sentence Intelligibility Test (SIT) developed by Yorkston, Beukelman and Tice (1996), are often used for clinical purposes in quantifying the severity of dysarthria (Ball, Willis, Beukelman, and Pattee, 2001; Hustad, 2008). A number of studies have been conducted on speech intelligibility in ALS (Ball et al., 2001; Ball et al., 2004; Klasner and Yorkston, 2005; Nishio and Niimi, 2000; Strong et al., 1999; Yorkston, Strand, Miller, Hillel, and Smith, 1993; Yorkston et al., 1996; Yorkston et al, 1999). These studies revealed that regardless of the ALS onset type (bulbar, spinal or mixed) a decrease in speaking rate will be evident before a decline in speech intelligibility is observed (Ball et al., 2001; Ball et al., 2004; Ball et al., 2005; Nishio and Niimi, 2000; Yorkston et al., 1993). It was however found that whilst individuals with spinal onset ALS may experience a gradual reduction in speaking rate over an extended period, for individuals with bulbar onset ALS this period may be relatively brief (Ball et al., 2001). Thus, despite the traditional focus on speech intelligibility, speaking rate appears to also an effective measure to predict the loss of functional speech of PALS (Beukelman et al., 2008). Both reduced speech intelligibility and speaking rate are thus significant factors in determining whether individuals are effective communicators (Ball et al., 2004).

Communication effectiveness is defined as the ability of an individual to produce a message that has the intended result (Burleson and Denton, 1997; Hustad, 1999). It therefore implies that an individual has an adequate level of communication to meet important communication goals (Light, 1989). Communication, by nature, is an interactive process that does not occur in universal situations but rather in specific contexts across a range of social communication situations characterized by personal communication purposes and circumstances (Tönsing, Alant, and Lloyd, 2005). Research has confirmed that both PALS and their familiar communication partners agree that adverse communication situtations (e.g. noisy environments or speaking for an extended period) are the most difficult for PALS and impacted on their communcation effectiveness (Ball et al., 2001; Ball et al., 2004).

The positive relationship between speech intelligibility, speaking rate and communication effectiveness in ALS has also been confirmed (Ball et al., 2004; Murphy, 2004). It has been reported that as a result of decreased communication function, in 80% of cases alternative communication strategies are required to support the daily communication needs of PALS and their family (Ball et al., 2004). Augmentative and alternative communication (AAC) is widely accepted among PALS and their families and is acknowledged as best practice (Beukelman, Ball and Fager, 2008; Fried-Oken et al., 2006). Regardless of the AAC strategies implemented, it is vital that the recommended strategies meet the changing physical needs of individuals as the disease progresses. These strategies should support multiple, adjustable access methods that allow individuals to transition from hand access to more sophisticated methods such as scanning, eye pointing or -tracking (Beukelman, Fager and Nordness, 2011). The use of AAC strategies can even in the face of profound motor deterioration preserve communication (Mathy et al. 2000). Communication is essential for the human experience and may in some cases be the single most important aspect for personal well-being (Light, 1997). Regardless of the degree of physical dependence, the ability to communicate empowers individuals to participate not only in their own care, but preserves some degree of control and psychological independence whilst still maintaining social networks (Lubinsky, 1997).

Social Roles

PALS may experience diverse losses as permanent physical and communication disability become part of everyday life (Katz, 2002). In the initial stages of the disease, activities and duties previously performed with ease might require modification and might eventually have to be abandoned as the disease progresses. These changes will predictably shatter the long-established roles that an individual performed on a daily basis and consequentially impose dramatic lifestyle changes (Fox and Sohlberg, 2000; Rolland, 1994).

The social roles adults perform in their daily life can be placed in the five broad categories of worker, student, citizen and leisurite, roles performed during recreation and leisure activities, and family member (Fox and Sohlberg, 2000). It is inevitable that participation in these roles may be impacted on with the onset of an acquired disability, as disability increases the amount of effort required to participate in these roles (Stuart, Lasker, and Beukelman, 2000).

One of the first roles that PALS has to relinquish is that of 'worker'. Decreased muscle strength and increased fatigue combined with progressive communication difficulties impede on their ability to successfully perform their daily work. This in turn leads to loss of income and position in society (Mathy et al., 2000). The opportunities to fulfil the roles of citizen, student and leisurite are also curtailed as they struggle to main independence in activities of daily living. Although important, these roles were found to be less important than fulfilling the role of family member (Brintnell, Madill, Montgomerie, and Stewin, 1992).

As symptoms increase and work and physical activities decrease, more importance is placed on interpersonal relationships (Young and McNicoll, 1998). However, it has been reported that the role of 'family member' is often most affected by an acquired disability (Fox and Sohlberg, 2000). As the functional aspects of the disability impinge on participation patterns within the family, new roles and responsibilities must be established within existing family relationships. The responsibility of financially supporting the family might shift to the spouse, the direct caregiving role of the mother with small children affected and children have to take over responsibilities previously fulfilled by the affected parent.

Adults with acquired communication disabilities anecdotally relate that their inability to fulfill communicative roles (e.g. within their roles of parent, friend and even patient) as the loss of access to life (Mathy et al., 2000). Social actitivies become increasingly limited as friends and family find it difficult to tolerate their reduced communication ability and subsequently decrease the time spent with them (Mathy et al., 2000). This exacerbates the social isolation these individuals already experience as a result of decreased physical abilities (McLeod and Clarke, 2007). The shift in responsibilities and excessive commitment to one role may be detrimental to the feelings of psychological well-being of the PALS (Fox and Sohlberg, 2000; McLeod and Clarke, 2007; Rolland, 1999; Ross and Deverell, 2004).

Psychosocial Impact

The psychosocial aspects of living with ALS have been explored in an extensive meta-analysis conducted by McLeod and Clarke (2007). The great psychological burden that accompanies the experience of ALS has been highlighted. A prevalence rate of between 11% and 15% has been reported for depression among PALS (Ganzini, Johnston, and Hoffman, 1999). Research has however found no evidence of direct association between the loss of physical ability in general and depression (Hillemacher, et al., 2004). Anxiety and levels of self-esteem were associated with the degree of physical disability and impact of illness on everyday functioning (Goldstein et al., 1998). It has been further been reported that persons with a chronic disabling condition may feel that they are a burden, despite family members' willingness and ability to provide support and help (Cutrona, 2004). The feelings of inadequacy, embarrassment, frustration and helplessness are often exacerbated by the presence of increasing communication difficulties (Lasker and Bedrosian, 2000; Mathy et al., 2000).

The progressively declining abilities in mobility, activities of daily living and communication experienced by PALS, greatly alters the life of the family (Cheung and Hocking, 2004; McLeod and Clarke, 2007; Savundranayagam, Hummert, and Montgomery, 2005).

Impact of ALS on the Marital Relationship

The diagnosis of ALS will predictably affect multiple aspects of the marital relationship. Spouses most often become the primary source of emotional support and direct physical care for PALS (Cutrona, 2004). Demands faced by spousal caregivers include taking care of financial expenses, the physical demands of direct care as well as the emotional demands (Kinsella, Cooper, Picton, and Murtagh, 1998). An increase in financial expenses is expected with the onset of ALS as the cost of medical care and assistive technology escalates in the presence of an often dwindling income when the PALS have to relinquish their employment.

The physical care demands on the spouse will increase as the disease progresses (Cutrona, 2004; Rolland, 1994). The well-spouse may be weighed down with the demands of taking over the ill-spouse's household duties and responsibilities (Ross and Deverell, 2004). Day to day routines may also be disrupted as new direct caregiving tasks evolve (Rolland, 1994). These physical care demands may over time impose dramatic lifestyle changes on the spouse who has to live with continual role changes and adjustment as the disease progresses (Cutrona, 2004; Fox and Sohlberg, 2000; Rolland, 1999).

The spouse also have to face the emotional demands of dealing with the concerns of their ill-partner as well as their own distress (Kinsella et al., 1998). The emotional demands experienced by spousal carers of individuals with multiple sclerosis include anxiety, depression, and reduced feelings of self-esteem (Cheung and Hocking, 2004). Feelings of social isolation increase as opportunities and time for leisure activities are restricted (Murray et al., 1997). Despite this, social support for caregivers is often lacking as family, friends and healthcare providers mostly focus on the person with chronic illness, negating the spouse's need for support and respite (Kowal et al., 2003; Murray et al., 1997).

It is thus evident that on an individual level both members of the couple will have to continually adjust to ALS. They will often report experiencing similar psychosocial effects as they deal with their own distress and that of their partner. The emotional trauma of the profound changes to their relationship often elicits strong emotions from both partners, including guilt, anger, resentment and frustration (Baikie, 2002; Ross and Deverell, 2004). Couples facing the stress of chronic illness must find ways to manage these emotions. One of the most effective and constructive ways of dealing with these emotions, is communication (Cutrona, 2004).

THE MODERATING EFFECT OF COMMUNICATION IN MARRIAGE

The central role that sensitive, open and direct communication plays in marriage should not be underestimated (Burleson and Denton, 1997). Of critical importance is the capability of spouses to listen to and understand each other, but also expressing themselves clearly and accurately (Beach and Arias, 1989; Navran, 1967). It has been reported that these abilities are essential for couples to cope with chronic illness (Cutrona, 1996; Ross and Deverell, 2004). Effective marital communication can be achieved through verbal (i.e. speech) and non-verbal communication (i.e. body language, gestures and facial expressions). The history of numerous shared conversations, allow spouses to become more sensitive to each other's non-verbal communication that will ultimately result in feelings of intense closeness (Kahn, 1970).

The importance of the positive relationship between communication and marital satisfaction is emphasized in the literature (Beach and Arias, 1989; Blais and Boisvert, 2007; Rhoades and Stocker, 2006). Couples that reported high marital satisfaction made superior use of both verbal and non-verbal communication that allow for the expression of emotions, thoughts and feelings (Beach and Arias, 1989).

Even under the best circumstances couples often fail to achieve successful communication. Research has indicated that it is reasonable to expect that damage to couples' ability to communicate effectively would negatively impact on their relationship with each other (Blais and Boisvert, 2007; Burleson and Denton, 1997; Cutrona, 2004).

Impact of Negative Life Events on Marital Communication

A negative life event, such as the onset of disability or illness, may disrupt the ability of couples to be functionally adequate in the communication (Blais and Boisvert, 2007). The communicative competence of couples, who are faced with ALS, is affected gradually as the disease progresses (Rolland, 2005). It is reported that the spouses of PALS experience psychological distress that correlates with their perceived loss of intimacy as predicted by changes in communication (Goldstein et al., 2002). In the early stages of ALS, PALS rely on residual speech to facilitate social closeness with their spouse; however as their communication impairment become more pronounced, multiple AAC strategies are used for this purpose (Beukelman and Yorkston, 1998; Fried-Oken, et al., 2006; Murphy, 2004).

Although much is known about the way in which PALS and their spouses are affected by onset of ALS, the changes that may occur in their relationship in the context of marriage have received minimal attention (O'Connor et al., 2008). Due to the dearth of information on the changes that occur in the marital relationship as a result of the declining speech intelligibility in PALS, the current study was conducted. It was postulated that the couples' perception of marital communication will decrease as the PALS speech intelligibility decline over the disease progression. Therefore, the primary aim of this study was to compare how PALS and their spouses perceive changes in their marital communication in relation to the deteriorating speech of PALS. The current study aimed first to describe the communication abilities and the speech intelligibility patterns of PALS: and second, the perception of marital communication indicated by couples across the disease progression.

METHODOLOGY

Research Design

A non-experimental correlational design was employed for this study. This design was selected as it is appropriate to examine the relationship between the deteriorating speech of PALS and the couple's perception of marital communication across the disease progression.

Participants

A non-probability, purposive sampling strategy was used to recruit participants for this study. The sample consisted of fourteen couples ($N = 28$) divided into two participant groups. The first participant group included PALS ($n_1 = 14$) and the second participant group their spouses ($n_2 = 14$).

Participant group 1: PALS. Fourteen participants with a neurologist confirmed diagnosis of ALS were included in this group. They were recruited with the assistance from the Motor Neuron Disease Association of South Africa (MNDSA) and met the following selection criteria: (i) had been in an established intimate relationship for at least 12 months prior to the onset of ALS; (ii) had no reported speech-language, hearing or visual impairment other that those resulting from the ALS. This group comprised 11 males and three females. Six participants presented with spinal onset ALS, six with bulbar onset ALS and two with mixed onset ALS. The average age of the participants was 57;1 (years; months) (range 44;1 to 70;4; *SD* = 8;67 years). The average time since the onset of the ALS symptoms was 3;76 (range 3 months to 8;6; *SD* = 2;19) and the average time since diagnosis was 2;37 (range 5 months to 7 years; *SD* = 2;08).

Of the fourteen participants, one participant was classified as having 'mild' ALS at the onset of the study, seven participants as 'moderate' and six as 'severe'. The disease progression was evident at the subsequent visits (See Figure 1). The attrition of participants as a result of death shortly after the second visit decreased the sample size to only nine participants at the final visit.

Participant group 2: Spouses. This group comprised the 14 spouses (n_2 = 14) of the PALS in participant group 1 (11 females and three males). None of these participants reported any communication, vision and hearing difficulties that impacted on their activities of daily living. The average age of the spouse group was 57;8 (range 47;6 to 70;3, *SD* = 8;64). The majority of the couples were married for more than a decade, with an average of 29;10 (range 3 years to 45;6, *SD* = 13;81).

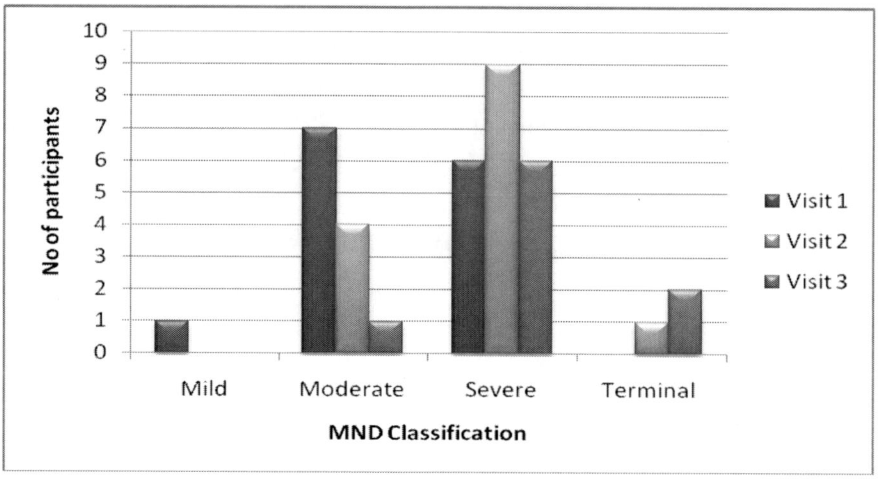

Figure 1. MND Classification across visits.

Materials

In order to meet the requirements pose by the research aims, five internationally accepted measures were utilized; Amyotrophic Lateral Sclerosis Severity Scale (ALSSS) (Hillel et al., 1989), Classification of MND (Riviere et al., 1998), Sentence Intelligibility Test (SIT) (Yorkston et al., 1996), Modified Communicative Effectiveness Index (CETI-M) (Yorkston, Beukelman, Strand and Bell, 1999) and the Primary Communication Inventory (PCI) (Navran, 1967).

Amyotrophic Lateral Sclerosis Severity Scale (ALSSS)

The severity level in the four categories of speech, swallowing, lower extremities and upper extremity abilities were determined using the ALSSS (Hillel et al., 1989). For the purposes of this study, only the results from the ALSSS speech scale is included to describe the functional impairment experienced by PALS participants in the area of speech. This scale includes five general categories namely normal speech processes, detectable speech disturbance, need for behavioural modifications, need for use of augmentative communication and loss of useful speech which is measured using a ten point scale of function.

Classification of MND

This classification system was developed by Riviere et al. (1998) to describe the ALS severity across the functional modalities of speech, mobility and the ability to use upper limbs for activities of daily living. Four states are indicated; mild (State 1), moderate (State 2), severe (State 3) and terminal (State 4).

Sentence Intelligibility Test

The SIT is a widely used standardised clinical transcription test (Yorkston et al., 1996). The SIT was used to objectively measure the speech intelligibility of PALS participants. Participants were required to read a series of 11 randomly generated, unrelated sentences varying in length of five to 15 words, at each visit. Using standard administration and measurement procedures, the transcription of recorded responses resulted in the percentage intelligibility productions.

Modified Communicative Effectiveness Index (CETI-M)

The CETI-M was adapted by Yorkston et al (1999) for the evaluation of the communicative effectiveness of PALS. Using a visual analogue scale, both PALS and their spouses were required to separately rate the PALS perceived communicative effectiveness across ten contextual situations on a seven point Likert scale.

Primary Communication Inventory

The Primary Communication Inventory (PCI) is a 25-item instrument designed to assess marital communication (Navran, 1967). The PCI was completed separately by both members of the couple at all three visits. It is reported that the overall score obtained by the PCI appears to be a reliable indicator of the soundness of communication between two members of a couple (Navran, 1967).

Procedures

Ethical approval for the study was obtained from the University Research Ethics Committee. Written informed consent was obtained from the MNDSA and all participants, using established and approved methods. All participants in the study were fully informed of the nature of the study and were assured of confidentiality and their right to withdraw from the study at any time, without any negative consequences. Participants were visited at home at times indicated as most convenient for both members of the couple. During the first visit, the aims of the research were explained and consent obtained. Demographic information was obtained from the couple, the ALSSS Speech Scale and Classification of MND was completed by the researcher based on the clinical observations and interviews with both members of the couple. The PALS completed the SIT, CETI-M and PCI with the assistance of the researcher. The spouses privately completed the CETI-M and PCI after receiving clear instructions. The two subsequent visits (visit 2 and visit 3) were scheduled at six-monthly intervals where the same measuring instruments as described for the first visit, were administered.

Reliability

The following basic considerations were taken into account during data collection. The recorded SIT responses were transcribed by the researcher using broad transcription techniques. The second rater, a speech-language pathologist unfamiliar with the participants and stimuli sentences, transcribed 25% of the SIT recordings. Interrater agreement for the SIT transcriptions was 95%.

Interrater agreement was also determined for the ALSSS, Classification of MND, CETI-M and PCI by the researcher and a second rater. The second rater, a registered nurse with 30-years clinical experience in the field of ALS, accompanied the researcher on 20% of the visits. At these visits she first determined the disease state according to the Classification of MND and then used clinical observation to rate the functional speech impairment of the PALS using the ALSSS Speech scale. She further independently completed the CETI-M and PCI while the first author conducted the interviews with the PALS. Across all these measurements the interrater agreement was 100%.

Data analysis and Statistical Procedures

Data was documented on all the relevant measuring instruments and encoded according to data definitions. Descriptive statistics were used to describe and analyse the data. The Friedman test was used with the repeated measures obtained from each participant group across the visits, whilst the Spearman rank correlation (*Rho*) was used to compute the correlation between speech intelligibility and communication effectiveness; as well as speech intelligibility and marital communication. The Wilcoxon test was used to compare the differences between the communication effectiveness ratings and marital communication scores of PALS and their spouses. In addition, Cohen's *d* (effect size) was calculated to establish the size of the statistically significant difference.

RESULTS

The purpose of this study was to compare how PALS and their spouses perceive changes in their marital communication in relation to the deteriorating speech of PALS. The current study aimed firstly to describe the communication abilities and the speech intelligibility patterns of PALS and secondly, the perception of marital communication indicated by couples across the disease progression.

Communication Abilities

The PALS participants' functional impairment in the area of speech was established with the ALSSS Speech Scale (Hillel et al., 1989). The progressive decline in speech function of participants with MND across all visits is evident. Seven participants reported 'detectable speech disturbances' at the first visit, five were required to make some 'behavioural modifications' and two used 'augmentative communication strategies' when communicating with both familiar and unfamiliar listeners. These two participants used a Lightwriter® a portable text-to-speech communication aid, to support communication with unfamiliar communication partners. Both participants operated the Lightwriter® by direct selection as they had adequate hand function. In addition to the Lightwriter®, they also implemented unaided low technology AAC strategies such as facial expression, head nodding and manual gestures and aided strategies such as alphabet boards (direct selection) to facilitate communication with their spouses.

The decline in speech intelligibility was evident at the second visit as only two participants indicated 'detectable speech disturbances'; while six were required to implement 'behavioural modifications', five made use of 'augmentative communication' and one reported 'loss of useful speech'. The participants who reported 'use of augmentative communication' mainly used unaided AAC strategies (such as facial expression and yes-or-no questions), aided low technology strategies (such as alphabet boards with optical direct selection using a laser pointing device attached to their head, and writing) to support their communication. One of the two participants who initially used a Lightwriter® for communication had to abandon use due to a significant decrease in hand function and mobility, making direct access to the Lightwriter® impossible. The participant who reported 'loss of useful speech' continued operating the Lightwriter® through direct selection for communication with unfamiliar listeners. He however preferred to use facial expression and manual gestures for communication with his spouse.

At the last visit only one participant reported a 'detectable speech disturbance', while three had to implement 'behavioural modifications', three used 'augmentative communication' and two reported 'loss of useful speech'. Participants who reported 'use of augmentative communication' and 'loss of useful speech' all facilitated communication with familiar and unfamiliar partners through facial expression, partner assisted yes-or-no questions, and/or direct optical selection alphabet boards. None of the participants made use of high technology AAC devices for communication at the last visit due to a decline in functional motor abilities.

Table 1. Speech intelligibility across visits

	Visit 1 $n = 14$	Visit 2 $n = 14$	Visit 3 $n = 9$
Mean	75.58 [a]	53.07 [ab]	36.22[b]
SD	22.93	32.81	24.6
Median	79.50	57.00	39.00
Cohen's *d*	0.9168 (large)		
Friedman *p*-value	0.0005*		

Mean with different superscript differ significantly at the 5% level.
* Significance at the 5% level.

Speech Intelligibility

The mean percentage speech intelligibility (as measured by the SIT) at the initial visit for all participants was 75.58% (range 35 to 100; *SD* = 22.93). At the second visit, the mean decreased to 53.07% (range 0 to 93; *SD* = 32.81) and finally to 36.22% (range 0 to 73; *SD* = 24.6) at the last visit. In order to determine whether the change in speech intelligibility was significant over time, a Friedman Test (two way analysis of variance) was employed (See Table 1). A statistically significant decrease in speech intelligibility was noted at the 5% confidence level between visits one and three and therefore the disease progression. Cohen's *d* (*d* = 0.9168) confirms that the effect of the difference between visit 1 and visit 3 is large (Cohen, 1992).

Communicative Effectiveness

The CETI-M (Yorkston et al., 1999) was used to describe the functional communication abilities of PALS across the disease progression.

Table 2. CETI-M ratings across visits and between participant groups

	Visit 1 $n = 14$ Mean	SD	Visit 2 $n = 14$ Mean	SD	Visit 3 $n = 9$ Mean	SD	Cohen's *d*	Friedman p – value
PALS	31.40 [a]	12.04	24.53 [ab]	10.25	21.00 [b]	6.84	0.5821**	0.0458*
Spouse	28.53 [a]	11.54	20.80 [ab]	9.74	18.77 [b]	9.30	0.6387**	0.0151*
Difference	0.6835		0.2812		0.1719			0.8948
Wilcoxon *p*-value	0.2578		0.0980		0.5078			

Mean with different superscript differs significantly at the 5% level.
* Significance at the 5% level.
** Between visit 1 and visit 3 – medium effect size.

Self-perceived effectiveness (as completed by PALS) and listener-perceived effectiveness (as completed by spouses) where obtained at each visit. Refer to Table 2 for a summary of the results obtained per participant group at each visit, the comparison over time for each group as well as the difference between the two groups.

A Friedman test was employed to determine whether the change in communicative effectiveness as rated by PALS and spouses was statistically significant over time. A *p*-value of 0.0458 was noted for PALS and 0.0151 for spouses, implying a significant decrease in communication effectiveness between visit 1 and visit 3. The effect size as measured with Cohen's *d* is medium for both participant groups (Cohen, 1992). The difference in CETI-M ratings between the two participant groups at each visit were determined by using a Wilcoxon test. As is evident in the *p*-values (0.2578, 0.0980 and 0.5078 respectively) no statistical significance at the 5% level was identified. A comparison of CETI-M ratings over time was determined by employing a Friedman Test. A *p*-value of 0.8948 was noted indicating no difference in ratings between the two participant groups over time.

Marital Communication

The second aim of the study, to describe the perception of marital communication as indicated by the couple across the disease progression, was addressed by administering the PCI at each visit to both participant groups. The possible range of scores that can be obtained on the PCI, is 25 to 125, with higher scores suggestive of more positively viewed marital communication The mean scores for 'happily' married couples are reported as 105 and 81 for 'unhappily' married couples (Navran, 1967).

A summary of the results obtained per participant group at each visit, the comparison over time for each group as well as the difference between the two groups are presented in Table 3. It is evident that the mean scores decreased across the visits. Although the scores were similar at the first visits, the decrease across visits was more apparent in the spouse participant group at the last two visits. Interesting, the mean PCI scores obtained at the first visit for both these groups were below 105, the mean score for 'happily' married couples.

A Friedman test was employed to determine whether the change in the perception of marital communication as rated by PALS and their spouses was statistically significant over time. A p-value of 0.8233 was noted for PALS implying that the change was not statistically significant. Contrary to these findings, the p-value obtained for spouses (0.0446) indicate a statistically significant decrease in perception of marital communication over time. Cohen's d confirms a medium effect size (d = 0.5562) between visit 1 and visit 3 (Cohen, 1992). No statistically significant difference was found between the PCI scores of the two participant groups between the visits and across the disease progression.

Table 3. Marital communication across visits and between participant groups

	Visit 1 $n = 14$		Visit 2 $n = 14$		Visit 3 $n = 9$		Cohen's d	Friedman p – value
	Mean	SD	Mean	SD	Mean	SD		
PALS	87.99	14.15	86.00	12.54	85.22	18.49	-	0.8233
Spouse	87.73	16.02	83.93	16.91	79.44	16.74	0.5562 **	0.0446*
Difference	0.9134		0.4966		0.5078			0.2359
Wilcoxon p-value	0.7763		0.6374		0.0576			

* Significance at the 5% level.
** Between visit 1 and visit 3 – medium effect size.

Speech Intelligibility and Marital Communication

Spearman's correlation was employed to compare whether PALS and their spouses perceive changes in their marital communication in relation to the deteriorating speech of PALS. Unexpectedly, no statistically significant correlations were found for either of the participant groups between speech intelligibility and marital communication.

DISCUSSION

Overall, the findings of this study prove that the assumption that communication between couples will invariably deteriorate as a result of progressively decreased speech intelligibility is not necessarily valid. The use of AAC can preserve the ability to develop and maintain intimate, rewarding relationships even in the face of profound physical disabilities (Prentice, 2000). The fundamental importance of communication in marriage is highlighted by Johnson (2000): "*Honest and effective communication is crucial for any healthy relationship and even more so when one of the partners is an augmented communicator*" (p. 47).

Predictably, compromised speech intelligibility limited verbal communication by PALS in this study. It is however postulated past shared experiences and familiarity often facilitates the spouse's ability to better interpret non-verbal communication such as gestures, vocalizations and facial expressions (Cutrona, 2004). Research highlights the importance that PALS place on the spouses' ability to understand communicative intent and meaning and therefore the maintenance of social closeness (Fried-Oken, et al., 2006; Murphy, 2004).

CONCLUSION

The current study was a preliminary effort to address the apparent dearth of information on the impact of progressive communication disabilities as a result of ALS on marital communication. A number of limitations in the study were however identified. The small sample size is the primary limitation of this study. The limited number of possible participants in South Africa, coupled with the unpredictable nature of ALS and the unique circumstances of individual couples negatively impacted on the sample size. The use of alternative statistical measures, such as Cohen's *d*, however, supports the notion that meaningful effect sizes moderate the need for larger sample sizes. Additionally, it is acknowledged that information about the marital relationship prior to the onset of ALS could have contributed to understanding the complexity of the each individual couple's unique relationship and the role that speech intelligibility plays in this regard.

Flowing from the above-mentioned limitations, it is recommended that this study is replicated using a larger sample size, preferably followed longitudinally. It is also suggested that prospective studies investigating the impact of speech intelligibility as a result of ALS on marital communication are conducted, as evidence suggests that the quality of the marital relationship prior to the onset of illness is a critical determinant of the extent to which chronic illness disrupts the marital relationship. The use of qualitative methods to explore these perceptions could offer invaluable insights in understanding of the impact of decreased communication abilities on marital relationships.

Communication as a means of facilitating and maintaining the marital relationship is particularly pertinent to PALS and their spouses. Health professionals should implement a holistic intervention approach that not only provide relief for the relentless physical deterioration, but also address the communication needs of PALS and their family. One of the most important clinical decisions is the appropriate timing of referrals to a speech therapist or AAC specialist for screening, assessment, intervention and education (Beukelman et al., 2011). It is essential to ensure that when residual speech is no longer effective, appropriate

AAC strategies are already in place that would encourage communication in all areas of life, but most specifically for the maintenance of social closeness within the marital relationship.

REFERENCES

Baikie, E. (2002). The impact of dementia on marital relationships. *Sexual and Relationships Therapy, 17* (3), 289-299.

Ball, L. J., Beukelman, D. R., and Pattee, G. L. (2004). Communication effectiveness of individuals with amyotrophic lateral sclerosis. *Journal of Communication Disorders, 37*, 197-215.

Ball, L. J., Beukelman, D. R., Ullman, C., Maassen, K., and Pattee, G. L. (2005). Monitoring speaking rate by telephone for persons with amyotrophic lateral sclerosis. *Journal of Medical Speech-Language Pathology, 13* (4), 233-238.

Ball, L. J., Willis, A., Beukelman, D. R., and Pattee, G. L. (2001). A protocol for the identification of early bulbar signs in amyotrophic lateral sclerosis. *Journal of the Neurological Sciences, 191* (1-2), 43-53.

Beach, S. H., and Arias, I. (1989). Assessment of perceptual discrepancy: Utility of the primary communication inventory. *Family Process, 22*, 309-316.

Beukelman, D. R., Ball, L. J., and Fager, S. (2008). An AAC personnel framework: Adults with acquired complex communication needs. *Augmentative and Alternative Communicatio, 24* (3), 255-267.

Beukelman D.M., Fager, S, and Nordness, A. (2011). Communication support for people with ALS. *Neurological Research International*, Article ID 714693, 6 pages. doi:10.1155/2011/714693.

Beukelman, D. R., and Yorkston, K. M. (1998). Augmentative and alternative communication application for persons with severe acquired communication disorders: An introduction. *Augmentative and Alternative Communication, 5* (1), 42-48.

Blais, M. C., and Boisvert, J. (2007). Psychological adjustment and marital satisfaction following head injury. Which critical personal characteristics should both partners develop? *Brain Injury, 21* (4), 357-372.

Brintnell, E. S., Madill, H. M., Montgomerie, T. C., and Stewin, L. L. (1992). Work and family after injury: Do female and male client perspectives differ? *Career Development Quarterly, 41*, 145-160.

Burleson, B. R., and Denton, W. H. (1997). The relationship between communication skill and marital satisfaction: Some moderating effects. *Journal of Marriage and the Family*, 59, 884-902.

Charmaz, K. (1995). The body, identity, and self: Adapting to impairment. *Sociological Quarterly, 36*(4), 657-681. http://search.proquest.com/ docview/200535741?accountid= 15083.

Cheung, J., and Hocking, P. (2004). Caring as worrying: The experience of spousal carers. *Journal of Advanced Nursing, 47* (5), 475-482.

Cohen, J. (1992). A power primer. *Psychological Bulletin, 112*, 155-159.

Cutrona, C. E. (2004). A psychological perspective: Marriage and the social provisions of relationships. *Journal of Marriage and Family, 66*, 992-999.

Darley, F., Aronson, A., and Brown, J. (1969). Clusters of deviant speech dimensions in the dysarthrias. *Journal of Speech and Hearing Disorders, 12*, 462-496.

Duffy, J. (1995). *Motor speech disorders: Substrates, differential diagnosis and management.* Baltimore: Mosby.

Fox, L. E., and Sohlberg, M. M. (2000). Meaningful communication roles. In D. R. Beukelman, K. M. Yorkston, and J. Reichle (Eds.), *Augmentative and alternative communication for adults with acquired neurological disorders* (pp. 3-24). Baltimore: Paul H. Brookes.

Fried-Oken, M., Fox, L., Rau, M. T., Tullman, J., Baker, G., Hindal, M., et al. (2006). Purposes of ACC device use for persons with ALS as reported by caregivers. *Augmentative and Alternative Communication, 22* (3), 209-221.

Ganzini, L., Johnston, W. S., and Hoffman, W. F. (1999). Correlates of suffering in amyotrophic lateral sclerosis. *Neurology, 52*, 1434-1440.

Goldstein, L. H., Adamson, M., Jeffrey, L., Down, K., Barby, T., Wilson, C., et al. (1998). The psychological impact of MND on patients and carers. *Journal of the Neurological Sciences, 160* (Suppl.1), S114-S121.

Hillel, A.D., Miller, R. M., Yorkston, K., McDonald, E., Norris, F.H., and Konikow, N. (1989). Amyotrophic lateral sclerosis severity scale. *Neuroepidemiology, 8* (3), 142-150.

Hillemacher, T., Gräβel, E., Tigges, S., Bleich, S., Neundörfer, B., Kornhuber, J., et al. (2004). Depression and bulbar involvement in amyotrophic lateral sclerosis. *ALS and other motor neuron disorders, 5*, 245-249.

Hustad, K. (1999). Optimizing communicative effectiveness. In K. M. Yorkston, D. R. Beukelman, E. A. Strand, and K. R. Bell (Eds.), *Management of motor speech disorders in children and adults* (2nd ed., pp. 483-542). Austin: ProEd.

Johnson, P. L. (2000). If I do say so myself. In M. Fried-Oken, and J. H. Bersani (Eds.), *Speaking up and spelling it out* (pp. 47-56). Maryland: Paul H. Brookes.

Kahn, M. (1970). Non-verbal communication and marital satisfaction. *Family Process, 9*, 449-456.

Katz, J. (2002). Ill-health. In N. Thompson (Ed.), *Loss and grief: A guide for human service practitioners* (pp. 149-161). Hampshire: Palgrave.

Kinsella, G., Cooper, B., Picton, C., and Murtagh, D. (1998). A review of the measurement of caregiver and family burden in palliative care. *Journal of Palliative Care, 14* (2), 37-45.

Kowal, J., Johnson, S. M., and Lee, A. (2003). Chronic illness in couples: A case for emotionally focused therapy. *Journal of Marital and Family Therapy, 29* (3), 299-310.

Kuhnlein, P., Gdynia, H.J., Sperfeld, A.D., Linder-Pfleghar, B., Ludolph, A.C., Prosiegel, M., and Riecker, A. (2008). Nature clinical practice neurology. Diagnosis and treatment of bulbar symptoms in ALS. *Amyotrophic Lateral Sclerosis, 4,* 366 - 374.

Lasker, J. P., and Bedrosian, J. L. (2000). Acceptance of AAC by adults with acquired disorders. In D. R. Beukelman, K. M. Yorkston, and J. Reichle (Eds.), *Augmentative and alternative communication for adults with acquired neurologic disorders* (pp. 107-136). Baltimore: Paul H. Brookes.

Leigh, P.N., Abrahams, S., Al-Chalabi, A., Ampong, M.A., Goldstein, L.H., Johnson, J., … Willey, E. (2003). The management of motor neuron disease. *Journal of Neurology, Neurosurgery and Psychiatry. 74,* 432 - 447.

Light, J. (1997). "Communication is the essence of human life": Reflections on communicative competence. *Augmentative and Alternative Communication, 13*, 61-70.

Light, J. C., Arnold, K. B., and Clark, E. A. (2003). Finding a place in the 'social circle of life'. In J. C. Light, D. R. Beukelman, and J. Reichle (Eds.), *Communicative competence for individuals who use AAC: From research to effective practice.* Baltimore: Paul H. Brookes Publishing Co.

Lubinsky, R. (1997). Perspectives on aging and communication. In R. Lubinsky, and D. J. Higginbothan (Eds.), *Communication technologies for the elderly: Vision, hearing and speech* (pp. 1-22). San Diego: Singular Publishing.

Mathy, P., Yorkston, K. M., and Gutmann, M. L. (2000). AAC for individuals with amyotrophic lateral sclerosis. In D. R. Beukelman, K. M. Yorkston, and J. Reichle (Eds.), *Augmentative and alternative communication for adults with acquired neurological disorders* (pp. 183-232). Baltimore: Paul H. Brookes.

McLeod, J. E., and Clarke, D. M. (2007). A review of psychosocial aspects of motor neurone disease. *Journal of the Neurological Sciences, 258*, 4-10.

Murphy, J. (2004). "I prefer contact this close": Perceptions of AAC by people with motor neuron disease and their communication partners. *Augmentative and Alternative Communication, 20*, 259-271.

Murray, J. M., Manela, M. V., Shuttleworth, A., and Livingston, G. A. (1997). Caring for an older spouse with psychiatric illness. *Aging and Mental Health, 1* (3), 256-260.

Navran, L. (1967). Communication and adjustment in marriage. *Family Process, 6*, 173-184.

Nishio, M., and Niimi, S. (2000). Changes over time in dysarthric patients with amyotrophic lateral sclerosis (ALS): A study of changes in speaking rate and maximum repetition rate (MRR). *Clinical Linguistics and Phonetics, 14* (7), 485-497.

O'Connor, E. J., McCabe, M. P., and Firth, L. (2008). The impact of neurological illness on marital relationships. *Journal of Sex and Marital Therapy, 34*, 115-132.

Rhoades, G. K., and Stocker, C. M. (2006). Can spouses provide knowledge of each other's communication patterns? A study of self-reports, spouses' reports, and observational coding. *Family Process, 45*, 499-511.

Riviere, M., Meininger, V., Zeisser, P., and Munsat, T. (1998). An analysis of extended survival in patients with amyotrophic lateral sclerosis treated with riluzole. *Archives of Neurology, 55* (4), 526-528.

Rolland, J. S. (1994). In sickness and in health: The impact of illness on couples' relationships. *Journal of Marital and Family Therapy, 20* (4), 327-343.

Rolland, J. S. (1999). Chronic illness and the family life cycle. In B. Carter, and M. McGoldrick (Eds.), *The expanded family life cycle: Individual, family, and social perspectives* (3rd ed., pp. 492-551). Needham Heights: Allyn and Bacon.

Ross, E., and Deverell, A. (2004). *Psychosocial approaches to health, illness and disability. A reader for health care professionals.* Pretoria: Van Schaik Publishers.

Tönsing, K. M., Alant, E., and Lloyd, L. L. (2005). Augmentative and alternative communication . In E. Alant, and L. L. Lloyd (Eds.), *Augmentative and alternative communication and severe disabilities: Beyond poverty* (pp. 30-67). London: Whurr Publishers.

Savundranayagam, M. Y., Hummert, M. L., and Montgomery, R. J. (2005). Investigating the effects of communication problems on caregiver burden. *The Journals of Gerontology, 60B* (1), S48-S55.

Strong, M. J., Grace, G. M., Orange, J. B., Leeper, H. A., Menon, R. S., and Aere, C. (1999). A prospective study of cognitive impairment in ALS. *Neurology, 53* (8), 1665-1670.

Stuart, S., Lasker, J. P., and Beukelman, D. R. (2000). AAC message management. In D. R. Beukelman, K. M. Yorkston, and J. Reichle (Eds.), *Augmentative and alternative communication for adults with acquired neurologic disorders* (pp. 25-54). Baltimore: Paul H. Brookes.

World Health Organization (2001). *International Classification of Functioning, Disability and Health (ICF).* Geneva: WHO Press.

Yorkston, K. M., Miller, R. M., and Strand, E. A. (1995). *Management of speech and swallowing disorders in degenerative disease.* Tuscon: Communication Skill Builders.

Yorkston, K. M., Beukelman, D. R., and Tice, R. (1996). *Sentence Intelligibility Test for Windows.* Lincoln: Institute for Rehabilitation Science and Engineering, Madonna Rehabilitation Hospital.

Yorkston, K. M., Beukelman, D. R., Strand, E. A., and Bell, K. R. (1999). *Management in motor speech disorders in children and adults* (2nd ed.). Austin: Pro-Ed.

Yorkston, K. M., Strand, E., Miller, R. M., Hillel, A. D., and Smith, K. (1993). Speech deterioration in amyotrophic lateral sclerosis: Implications for the timing of intervention. *Journal of Medical Speech-Language Pathology, 1* (1), 35-46.

Young, J. M., and McNicoll, P. (1998). Against all odds: positive life experiences of people with advanced amyotrophic lateral sclerosis. *Health and Social Work, 23*, 35-43.

Yunusova, Y., Weismer, G., Kent, R. D., and Rusche, N. M. (2005). Breath-group intelligibiity in dysarthria: Characteristics and underlying correlates. *Journal of Speech, Language and Hearing Research, 48* (6), 1294-1310.

In: Amyotrophic Lateral Sclerosis
Editors: Katashi Segawa and Ryota Ijichi
ISBN: 978-1-62257-679-1

Chapter 5

Psychological Interventions in Amyotrophic Lateral Sclerosis

Francesco Pagnini[1,2]
[1] Department of Psychology, Catholic University of Milan, Italy
[2] NeuroMuscular Omnicentre, Niguarda Ca' Granda Hospital, Milan, Italy

Abstract

There are many psychological issues relevant to Amyotrophic Lateral Sclerosis. The progressive and currently un-stoppable nature of the disease may lead to a reaction that includes a depressive response, hopelessness and anxiety, in both ALS patients and caregivers. In a multidisciplinary ALS team, attention to psychological aspects can significantly improve the quality of life of patients and relatives. Psychologists may play an important role in care, from a bio-psycho-social perspective.

An initial psychological intervention may begin during the diagnosis phase, supporting the communication given by the physician, with attention to emotive and psychosocial aspects. After the diagnosis and during disease progression, patients and carers should be able to access a "safe place", a relationship with a professional where they can receive counselling, aimed at improving coping methods. Psychologists can increase the acceptance rate of devices such as wheelchairs, NIVs and communicators or, at least, promote a better awareness of their psychological significance. Specific counselling could be provided in the choice of invasive interventions, such as PEG of tracheostomy, and may be useful in the acceptance of end-of-life deliberations. Spiritual assistance, not strictly related to religious believes, can be very helpful to patients and their close relatives.

Psychological support may also be helpful for physicians, giving their burden of care. People who work with ALS patients are at a high risk of professional burnout. Psychological counselling may be an appropriate response to reduce this risk.

INTRODUCTION

Amyotrophic lateral sclerosis (ALS) is a progressive and fatal neurodegenerative disease that is clinically characterised by progressive weakness, leading to death by respiratory insufficiency usually within three years (Haverkamp, Appel, & Appel, 1995). ALS typically presents as muscle wasting or weakness in a limb or bulbar regions (Talbot, 2002). It then progresses to pervasive muscle weakness with a combination of upper and lower motor neuron dysfunction. Patients become immobile, develop impaired speech, and this often leads to social isolation. In late stages of the disease progressing paralysis can result in a "locked-in" state in which only residual muscular movement is possible (Mitchell & Borasio, 2007). So far it is not possible to prevent progression of the disease.

The incidence of ALS is reported to be between 1.5 and 2.7 per 100,000 population/year (average 1.89 per 100,000/year) in Europe and North America, with a uniform incidence across these countries (Worms, 2001). The mean age of onset for ALS is between 55 - 65 years, with 5 % of cases having an onset before the age of 30 years (Haverkamp, et al., 1995). Although most cases of ALS are sporadic, about 5 % of cases have a family history of ALS (Mulder, Kurland, Offord, & Beard, 1986).

The psychological impact of ALS may be huge, for both the patients and their families (Pagnini, In press). People with a diagnosis of ALS face two main issues: the lack of treatment to stop the progression of the illness that will lead to death within a few years and the progressive loss of physical functions, sometimes with underestimated pain experiences (Pagnini, et al., In press). These two main issues also have an impact on ALS caregivers.

Amyotrophic Lateral Sclerosis is also a challenge for physicians and carers who attempt to cure or take care of patients (Hardiman, Van Den Berg, & Kiernan, 2011). Death is a very present issue and coping with it is not easy. There are many psychoanalytic scholars who suggest that death is the final cause of human fears. Therefore, working closely to people with a condition that presents them with death, can be a cause of burnout for medical professions.

Considering that there are no available treatments to stop the progression of the disease, the primary goal in caring for patients with ALS is often considered to be the enhancement of their quality of life (Simmons, 2005). Quality of life (QoL) is generally defined in terms of bio-psycho-social issues, integrating physical and biological aspects (i.e. symptoms of an illness or wellness), psychological aspects (i.e. emotions and thoughts) and social aspects (i.e. family relationships and social support) (Engel, 1977).

Clinical evolution of ALS is similar in all patients, but loss of functions are different in their time of onset and speed of progression. Given the devastating nature of the disease, access to psychological support can be very important. As for other serious illnesses (i.e. cancer), psychological support should provide a supporting role, giving a safe emotional space where people can express their feelings and emotions, and be accompanied through the journey of their pain and fears. Psychologists can be very active in the rehabilitation process of ALS patients and they can provide specific support through every phase of disease progression.

Furthermore, psychologists should help not only the patient and family to understand what is happening, but also support other members of the multi-professional team in their attempt to manage the often complex situation in which they are involved. Even though there are many psychologists in the world who support people with ALS, there are few studies that have investigated psychological and psychotherapeutic interventions in this field (Pagnini, Simmons, Corbo, & Molinari, 2012). The present chapter is an expression of clinical experience, combined with first-hand evidence from research literature, and taking into account other chronic clinical situations.

IMMEDIATELY FOLLOWING DIAGNOSIS

The way in which ALS diagnosis is communicated to the patient is very important in determining their initial reaction (Simmons, 2005). The communication of the ALS diagnosis may cause major repeated psychological trauma which the patient will have to cope with (defence and adaptation mechanisms). Clinical management of ALS should include knowledge, understanding and acceptance of these mechanisms. This is a challenge for physicians, being that may be unprepared to break bad news (Buckman, 1996), probably due to a lack of emotional management training (Pagnini, Manzoni, & Castelnuovo, 2009). Guidelines for breaking the news to a patient with ALS do reference the chance to access psychological support (Borasio, Sloan, & Pongratz, 1998).

ALS diagnosis is a devastating label. It is something that will definitely change the patient's (and relatives') life and will provide a shorter life horizon. The perception of the approach of this horizon forces the person to face issues surrounding death. Immediately after diagnosis, patients often need a "space" in which they can express their emotions, usually their despair, concerning the illness they have just been diagnosed with.

As mentioned above, diagnostic communication of illness is a very important and emotionally relevant moment for the patient. The presence of a psychologist among clinical staff can help the patient to express their feelings and their fears better than to a physician. A patient-centred service should be very careful in diagnostic communication and the clinical team should work together to enhance the quality of the patient/clinician relationship, in particular during diagnostic and prognostic communication processes.

Relatives and caregivers of ALS patients should be able to receive psychological support immediately following diagnosis of the disease. The label "ALS" is a very heavy burden to carry, both for patients and their relatives. At the beginning, they need to cope with bereavement, caused by the knowledge of loss of functions, and by the awareness that, within a few years, the patient will probably die.

Psychological support for families is very important immediately after the diagnosis. During clinical interview, patients and carers should be able to express their fears and worries. One of the most helpful therapeutic elements that can be provided is active listening. There can be very long silences that express fear, pain and suffering. It is not easy for the professional to "stay" with the silence and the emotions expressed, because empathy mechanisms promote the development of similar suffering in the person listening. However, the result justifies the effort. Some of the most significant moments of the "talking cure" include no talking (Lane, Koetting, & Bishop, 2002). When the psychologist "listens" to the silence of the patient, the latter has the chance to explore emotions, rather than avoid them. Furthermore, the patient can feel as though they are accompanied by the psychologist and therefore they are not alone in the facing of painful experiences. It is not difficult to imagine how this can be important for ALS patients, who will be forced to remain in silence by the progress of the disease, and forced to face their inner world alone.

PSYCHOLOGICAL CONSULTATIONS DURING DISEASE PROGRESSION

During progression of the illness, psychological consultations can be both expressive, promoting mourning management, and practical, providing help through discussions and practical suggestions. Being aware of the existence of an emotionally safe place, provided by the psychologist, is a great resource for ALS patients, and significantly improving their quality of life. During counselling they can explore their needs, feel free to give voice to their emotions, which will have a cathartic effect. People can be seen on their own, in couple or as family. It is also possible to address practical troubles that cause personal, family or social diseases. Not all of these problems are necessarily related to the symptoms of ALS. Sometimes clinicians need to face pre-existing diseases, for example relationship problems in a couple, that are exacerbated by the new medical condition. Psychometric instruments can represent a valuable assistance to understand the level of psychological sufferance. In particular, the ALS-Specific Quality of Life Questionnaire (Simmons, et al., 2006) and the Hospital Anxiety and Depression Scale (Gibbons, et al., 2011) can provide interesting clinical information from patient's point of view.

Practical suggestions may be provided whenever a psychosocial or educational intervention is required. For example, patients and relatives can be worried and confused about "if" and "how" to communicate information about the disease to their small children and this could be an object of practical analysis in psychological counselling.

Throughout the course of the disease, physicians should learn how to maintain a balance between anticipating the onset of loss of functions and introducing life support measures on one hand, and respecting the patient's psychological state, life plans and environment on the other. The psychologist and other clinicians should have a strong cooperative activity, with two-way communications: the psychologist should provide information concerning the psychological well-being, acceptance rate and social issues of the patients, while medical staff should provide information about the clinical and functional level of the patient. Multi-disciplinary teams should hold discussions on a case-by-case basis with constant updates. Typically, team meetings are conducted at least once a week, with the presence of all involved professionals (Van den Berg, et al., 2005), including neurologists, pneumologists, physiatrists, psychologists, nurses, physiotherapists etc..

As the disease progresses, physical functions will decrease. Currently, medical knowledge is unable to reverse this process but can offer the use of auxiliaries to compensate, for instance: walkers, manual wheelchairs, or powered wheelchairs. Many people look at these auxiliaries as a "painful goodbye" to their autonomy, a limitation of freedom. These objects represent the loss of functions and, for some people, a "defeat" by the illness, in a battle that will never be won. On the other hand, the use of, for example, a wheelchair can provide many opportunities to the patient and can partially restore lost autonomy, without there being the strict dependence from other people for motility. In a dedicated interview, the psychologist could discussion these positive points if the patient expresses some resistance towards the use of these instruments. However, feelings and fears of becoming more and more dependent should be listened to and, whenever possible, the clinician should promote positive management.

Furthermore, ALS patients will, sooner or later, face loss of speech and voice. An initial decrease of speech volume is common, followed by a change in voice, becoming more confused. This may be followed by complete loss of speech. Communication problems can be psychologically and socially devastating. The inability to communicate can make patients feel isolated and, moreover, the lack of ability to express their emotions and feelings has been reported as a distressing experience in different situations (Kerns, Rosenberg, & Jacob, 1994). From the carers' point of view, it can be even more difficult to understand the needs of the patient, sometimes with an increased burden and psychological sufferance. However, speech is not the only way in which it is possible to communicate. In order to prevent negative psychological and social consequences, patients and caregivers should access other forms of communication. In addition to technological solutions, such as computerised communicators, there are a lot of possible ways to communicate, like hand signals, head nodding and sign language (Simmons, 2005). Psychologists should facilitate the awareness that living without speech is not living without communication. Furthermore, it is essential that the caregiver/patient partnership finds a way to communicate easily between them, according to the specific situation and relationship.

At a certain stage of the illness, ALS patients' respiratory capacity will begin to decrease. Ventilatory ability worsens, providing a reduction in oxygen availability. Respiratory support is usually provided by Non Invasive Ventilation (NIV) or invasive ventilation via tracheotomy. NIV is the provision of ventilatory support through the patient's upper airway using a mask or similar device, while tracheotomy is a surgical procedure on the neck to open a direct airway through an incision in the trachea. NIV is usually initially used for sporadic nocturnal support to alleviate symptoms of nocturnal hypoventilation. As respiratory function worsens, patients tend to require increasing daytime NIV support and eventually continuous support.

Together with emotional strain from the decrease in respiratory functions, many patients report a rejection of the mask, describing an experience similar to claustrophobia, where they feel suffocated and increasing anxiety and anguish. The psychologist can allow a controlled expression of these feelings, reducing anxious symptomatology. Relaxation techniques can be useful against this phobia and the related anxiety (Manzoni, Pagnini, Castelnuovo, & Molinari, 2008). In particular, the use of systematic desensitisation can be helpful in the improvement of mask acceptance. Systematic desensitisation (Wolpe, 1990) is a technique used to treat phobias and other extreme or erroneous fears based on principles of behaviour modification. After learning relaxation skills, the anxious trigger, such as the mask, is gradually introduced as the anxiety-provoking stimuli. At first, it is possible to imagine the mask and imagine that it is gradually getting closer. When the patient is relaxed with the image of the mask being placed on the face, it is possible to gradually introduce the real mask, with different steps of distance and time of ventilation (from a few seconds to more than several hours required for ventilation therapy).

Bulbar dysfunctions lead to a risk of malnutrition and dehydration. Nutrition troubles in ALS usually begin with thin liquids and then progresses to involve food of other consistencies. The patient's capacity to swallow food decreases as the tongue weakens and coughing and choking increase. Management of dysphagia initially consists of recommendations of changes in food consistency, but when these methods are not enough, it is usually proposed that a feeding gastrostomy tube be introduced to the patient (PEG or RIG). Food has many symbolic and psychological meanings that are not easily summarised. Therefore, it is important to explore the subjective meaning that the patient prescribes to the inability to eat. For some people it can even represent a narcissistic wound because eating some food could have been part of their identity.

Despite variety in disease progression, sooner or later all ALS patients must face important decisions. In particular, choices about nutrition management or addressing breathing problems with a tracheostomy.

These choices are very important and hard to take because of the impact on their lives. Patients should be able to make a choice being conscious of the medical issues, communicated by physicians, but also given time to express their fears and doubts. When the patient takes a decision about an intervention an informed consent must be signed. Banfi and colleagues (Banfi, et al., 2009) proposed a two-step informed consent, with communication of clinically relevant information by the physician and a second phase, after hours or even days, when a patient can explore feelings and fears with a psychologist. Only in this second phase will the consent be signed.

End-of-Life Phase

In the final phase of the disease, physical impairments restrict the patient to remaining lying in bed, with limited abilities to move and communicate with others. This is often labelled as the "end-of-life" phase. The approach of the end of the life, death, often leads to fears, grief and sadness, in both patients and the people around them. Psychological support becomes even more important in this phase of disease.

Psychologists need to be aware of potential difficulties in bereavement outcome for surviving relatives and for carers. Difficult questions are often asked of clinicians, related to the management of suffering at the end of life, from both patients and caregivers. Emotional strain in this period is very high and can promote psychological diseases in pre-morbid subjects. There could be requests for assistance in dying, as a means of stopping the suffering. Answers to these questions should be given sensitively and honestly, considering the ability of the individual to understand and manage the information that they are requesting.

After a patient's death, continuous counselling is often needed in order to cope with the grief of mourning. The death of a person has a lasting effect on their family and not all people are able to cope well with the situation (Martin & Turnbull, 2001). Grief and bereavement support is integral to ALS care, but a study conducted in the US indicate that the support provided by ALS centres is often inadequate (Hebert, Lacomis, Easter). Measures such as a letter of condolence and the availability of a psychologist to talk to can improve this support. A letter of condolence can help a bereaved family and tie-up the relationship between the physician and the family (Bedell, Cadenhead, & Graboys, 2001).

THE HEALING ROLE OF SPIRITUALITY AND RELIGIOUSNESS

Spirituality can been defined as a search for the sacred or divine through any life experience (National Institute for Healthcare Research, 1997), but a broader definition would include feelings of connectedness with the self, a community, nature, and the meaning or purpose of life (Bellingham, Cohen, Jones, & Spaniol le, 1989). The concept of spirituality is similar, but not identical to, the concept of religion. The term "religious" often relates to a person's adherence to the beliefs, values and practices proposed by an organised institution which is devoted to the search for the divine through prescribed ways of viewing and living life (Thoresen, 1998). Researchers often use these terms interchangeably, which may lead to confusion. Religion and spirituality are not mutually exclusive concepts and can overlap and exist separately and are both very important, often underestimated, issues in health care (Lambert, 2006).

ALS patients often describe their spiritual beliefs as providing a profound method of coping with the disease and improving their quality of life (Pagnini, Rossi, Lunetta, Banfi, & Corbo, 2010). Spirituality and existential well-being issues should be addressed and explored in interviews, with respect and the awareness that they are very powerful resources in coping with illness and the shadow of death. Spirituality and attitude toward religious believes can be a great source of strength for patients, their caregivers (Pagnini, et al., 2011) and the psychologist that is providing the support. It can provide a sense of meaning about the illness and, more in general, about life. This sense of meaning is one of the few issues that may contrast the feeling of desperation related to the awareness of death approaching. For these reasons, it is sometimes useful for psychologists to send patients to a spiritual counsellor, according to their believes (i.e. a priest, a monk or maybe a philosopher).

Further studies concerning these issues and their positive consequences on ALS patients and carers should be encouraged.

TAKING CARE OF THE CAREGIVERS

The burden experienced by ALS caregivers is severe, as for caring for sufferers of any neurological disorder (Pagnini, Rossi, Lunetta, Banfi, Castelnuovo, et al., 2010). Hecht and colleagues (Hecht, et al., 2003) analysed the burden of ALS carers, comparing it to that experienced by carers of other diseases. They found that the level of care burden for ALS was low compared with dementia, mixed neuropsychiatric and internal diseases, but it correlated with functional impairment. Personal and social restrictions, and physical and emotional problems were the main burden components. Given that the burden of care increases with functional impairment, these researchers suggest that support for caregivers has to start sooner.

Caregivers spend a lot of time caring, sometimes more than 11 hours a day, despite having other assistance in the home (Krivickas, Shockley, & Mitsumoto, 1997) and those who believe they cannot leave the patient are the most distressed (Rabkin, Wagner, & Del Bene, 2000).

Together with emotional strain, care in ALS requires a certain amount of physical effort, in particular during the advanced phases of the disease. Patients need assistance in movement and to get up, and it could be a problem for people with physical impairments. This is particularly true for older caregivers, who may have their own age-related troubles (Pagnini, Lunetta, et al., 2012).

The progressive nature of the disease promotes dependence of the patient upon a primary caregiver and it is important to identify factors relevant to quality of life for both patient and caregiver (Lo Coco, et al., 2005) and to improve these as much as possible. There is some evidence supporting the idea that caregivers influence the mental and physical status of patients with ALS (Chio, Gauthier, Calvo, Ghiglione, & Mutani, 2005). The therapeutic team should be aware of the strengths and deficiencies of the caregivers, and should help them in improving their coping skills. Since concordance of depression and distress levels between patients and caregivers is high, attention to the mental health of the caregiver could alleviate the patient's distress as well (Rabkin, et al., 2000).

Caregivers may benefit from psychological support, sometimes even more than the patient. Even if caregivers are aware of their psychological sufferance, sometimes it can be difficult to engage with them in continuing psychological support as they emphasis that it is the relative with ALS who is in need of counselling. Sometimes, they believe that they're shirking their duty if they get someone in to help. However, clinicians should communicate the message that if they want to provide good care to their disabled relative then they must take care of themselves, in the same way in which airline attendants instruct passengers traveling with children to put their oxygen mask on first if cabin air pressure falls so that they can most effectively help their children. Clinicians can support the caregiver in many ways, from psychological education at the beginning of the illness, to psychological support after the patient's death. Apart from psychological counselling, it is important that the clinical team acknowledges the difficulties that they are experiencing, with encouragement and appreciation.

Perceived social support is an important predictor of carer distress (Goldstein, Atkins, Landau, Brown, & Leigh, 2006), marital relationship satisfaction (O'Connor E, McCabe, & Firth, 2008) and patient's quality of life (Gauthier, et al., 2007). However, maintenance of a network of social support may be difficult to accomplish, as friends often stop visiting or became awkward around the patient as symptoms increase in severity (Cobb & Hamera, 1986). Even if the enhancement of relationships may be considered as a task for other specialists, the clinician can work with caregivers and patients in order to improve their social networks as this could have a positive influence on their QoL.

CONCLUSION

Many psychological reactions can arise when people are forced to face ALS. Depressive features, grief, sufferance, anxiety and the care burdening are common symptoms of ALS patients and their caregivers. Clinical staff are also at risk of burnout, given their empathic closeness to psychological sufferance and the lack of a definitive cure for the illness. Therefore, taking care of ALS patients may be difficult for physicians and other health professionals. Physicians need to accept that their interventions will not be able to reverse the course of the disease and, therefore, they will not be able to "save the patient's life". The awareness that their work can "only" slow down the disease progression can sometimes be a heavy burden to be carried by the physician. Multidisciplinary meetings, or even Balint groups (Kjeldmand & Holmstroem, 2008), with the presence of psychologists and physicians, can be of support to the clinical team and help prevent burnout.

As presented in this chapter, there is a lot of work to do for a psychologist in ALS care. During the entire progression of the disease, ALS patients, caregivers and also clinicians may experience many psychological reactions, that sometimes need to be addressed with a professional consultation. The variety of thoughts and emotions, together with the intensity of feelings, suggests that the consultation should be provided by an expert psychologist, with a wide knowledge of psychological theories and techniques. The closeness to sufferance requires a personal involvement and is a challenge for every clinician. Supervision and peer consultations could be useful tools, especially at the beginning of work in the ALS field, and the maintenance of attention toward their own needs and feelings is always essential. Psychologists should consider the oxygen mask metaphor not only for caregivers, but also for themselves.

Acknowledgment

The paper was developed in the mainframe of the project "Mindfulness-Based Cognitive Therapy for patients with Amyotrophic Lateral Sclerosis: a Randomized Controlled Trial", financed by the Italian Ministry of Health, Young Researcher Call 2009, project code GR-2009-1607388.

References

Banfi, P., Rossi, G., Pagnini, F., Cellotto, N., Gorni, K. O., Lunetta, C., et al. (2009). [Towards a multi-step informed consent: considerations and proposals for a good practice]. *La Clinica Terapeutica, 160*(6), 425-426.

Bedell, S. E., Cadenhead, K., & Graboys, T. B. (2001). The doctor's letter of condolence. *New England Journal of Medicine 344*(15), 1162-1164.

Bellingham, R., Cohen, B., Jones, T., & Spaniol le, R. (1989). Connectedness: some skills for spiritual health. *American Jounal of Health Promotion, 4*(1), 18-31. doi: 10.4278/0890-1171-4.1.18.

Borasio, G. D., Sloan, R., & Pongratz, D. E. (1998). Breaking the news in amyotrophic lateral sclerosis. *Journal of Neurological Science, 160*(Suppl 1), S127-133.

Buckman, R. (1996). Talking to patients about cancer. *BMJ, 313*(7059), 699-700.

Chio, A., Gauthier, A., Calvo, A., Ghiglione, P., & Mutani, R. (2005). Caregiver burden and patients' perception of being a burden in ALS. *Neurology, 64*(10), 1780-1782. doi: 64/10/1780 [pii] 10.1212/01.WNL.0000162034.06268.37.

Cobb, A. K., & Hamera, E. (1986). Illness experience in a chronic disease – ALS. *Social Science and Medicine, 23*, 641-650.

Engel, G. L. (1977). The need for a new medical model: a challenge for biomedicine. *Science, 196*(4286), 129-136.

Gauthier, A., Vignola, A., Calvo, A., Cavallo, E., Moglia, C., Sellitti, L., et al. (2007). A longitudinal study on quality of life and depression in ALS patient-caregiver couples. *Neurology, 68*(12), 923-926. doi: 68/12/923 [pii] 10.1212/01.wnl.0000257093.53430.a8.

Gibbons, C. J., Mills, R. J., Thornton, E. W., Ealing, J., Mitchell, J. D., Shaw, P. J., et al. (2011). Rasch analysis of the hospital anxiety and depression scale (hads) for use in motor neurone disease. *Health and Quality of Life Outcomes, 9*.

Goldstein, L. H., Atkins, L., Landau, S., Brown, R., & Leigh, P. N. A. M. (2006). Predictors of psychological distress in carers of people with amyotrophic lateral sclerosis: a longitudinal study. *Psychological Medicine, 36*(6), 865-875. doi: S0033291706007124 [pii] 10.1017/S0033291706007124.

Hardiman, O., Van Den Berg, L. H., & Kiernan, M. C. (2011). Clinical diagnosis and management of amyotrophic lateral sclerosis. *Nature Reviews Neurology, 7*(11), 639-649.

Haverkamp, L. J., Appel, V., & Appel, S. H. (1995). Natural history of amyotrophic lateral sclerosis in a database population. Validation of a scoring system and a model for survival prediction. *Brain, 118 (Pt 3)*, 707-719.

Hebert, R. S., Lacomis, D., Easter, C., Frick, V., & Shear, M. K. (2005). Grief support for informal caregivers of patients with ALS: a national survey. *Neurology, 64*(1), 137-138. doi: 64/1/137 [pii] 10.1212/01.WNL.0000148586.79290.A6.

Hecht, M. J., Graesel, E., Tigges, S., Hillemacher, T., Winterholler, M., Hilz, M. J., et al. (2003). Burden of care in amyotrophic lateral sclerosis. *Palliative Medicine, 17*(4), 327-333.

Kerns, R. D., Rosenberg, R., & Jacob, M. C. (1994). Anger expression and chronic pain. *Journal of Behavioral Medicine, 17*(1), 57-67.

Kjeldmand, D., & Holmstroem, I. (2008). Balint groups as a means to increase job satisfaction and prevent burnout among general practitioners. *Annals of Family Medicine, 6*(2), 138-145. doi: Doi 10.1370/Afm.813.

Krivickas, L. S., Shockley, L., & Mitsumoto, H. (1997). Home care of patients with amyotrophic lateral sclerosis (ALS). *Journal of the Neurological Sciences, 152 Suppl 1*, S82-89.

Lambert, R. (2006). Spiritual care. In D. Oliver, G. D. Borasio & D. Walsh (Eds.), *Palliative care in amyotrophic lateral sclerosis: from diagnosis to bereavement, 2nd edn*. Oxford: Oxford University Press.

Lane, R. C., Koetting, M. G., & Bishop, J. (2002). Silence as communication in psychodynamic psychotherapy. *Clinical Psychology Review, 22*(7), 1091-1104. doi: 10.1016/s0272-7358(02)00144-7.

Lo Coco, G., Lo Coco, D., Cicero, V., Oliveri, A., Lo Verso, G., Piccoli, F., et al. (2005). Individual and health-related quality of life assessment in amyotrophic lateral sclerosis patients and their caregivers. *Journal of the Neurological Sciences, 238*(1-2), 11-17. doi: S0022-510X(05)00228-5 [pii] 10.1016/j.jns.2005.05.018.

Manzoni, G. M., Pagnini, F., Castelnuovo, G., & Molinari, E. (2008). Relaxation training for anxiety: a ten-years systematic review with meta-analysis. *BMC Psychiatry, 8*, 41. doi: 1471-244X-8-41 [pii] 10.1186/1471-244X-8-41.

Martin, J., & Turnbull, J. (2001). Lasting impact in families after death from ALS. *Amyotrophic Lateral Sclerosis, 2*(4), 181-187. doi: 10.1080/14660820152882188 TQFATRWEVBYT1NY4 [pii]

Mitchell, J. D., & Borasio, G. D. (2007). Amyotrophic lateral sclerosis. *Lancet, 369*(9578), 2031-2041. doi: S0140-6736(07)60944-1 [pii] 10.1016/S0140-6736(07)60944-1.

Mulder, D. W., Kurland, L. T., Offord, K. P., & Beard, C. M. (1986). Familial adult motor neuron disease: amyotrophic lateral sclerosis. *Neurology, 36*(4), 511-517.

National Institute for Healthcare Research. (1997). *Final Report. Scientific Progress in Spiritual Research*. Rockville, MD: NIHR.

O'Connor E, J., McCabe, M. P., & Firth, L. (2008). The impact of neurological illness on marital relationships. *Journal of Sex & Marital Therapy, 34*(2), 115-132. doi: 789999340 [pii] 10.1080/00926230701636189.

Pagnini, F. (In press). Psychological well-being and quality of life in Amyotrophic Lateral Sclerosis: a review. *International Journal of Psychology*.

Pagnini, F., Lunetta, C., Banfi, P., Rossi, G., Fossati, F., Marconi, A., et al. (In press). Pain in Amyotrophic Lateral Sclerosis: a psychological perspective. *Neurological Sciences*. doi: 10.1007/s10072-011-0888-6.

Pagnini, F., Lunetta, C., Banfi, P., Rossi, G., Gorni, K., Castelnuovo, G., et al. (2012). Anxiety and Depression in Patients with Amyotrophic Lateral Sclerosis and Their Caregivers. *Current Psychology, 31*(1), 79-87.

Pagnini, F., Lunetta, C., Rossi, G., Banfi, P., Gorni, K., Cellotto, N., et al. (2011). Existential well-being and spirituality of individuals with amyotrophic lateral sclerosis is related to psychological well-being of their caregivers. *Amyotrophic Lateral Sclerosis, 12*(2), 105-108. doi: 10.3109/17482968.2010.502941.

Pagnini, F., Manzoni, G. M., & Castelnuovo, G. (2009). Emotional Intelligence Training and Evaluation in Physicians. *Jama-Journal of the American Medical Association, 301*(6), 600-600.

Pagnini, F., Rossi, G., Lunetta, C., Banfi, P., Castelnuovo, G., Corbo, M., et al. (2010). Burden, depression, and anxiety in caregivers of people with amyotrophic lateral sclerosis. *Psychology, Health & Medicine, 15*(6), 685-693. doi: 930872255 [pii] 10.1080/13548506.2010.507773.

Pagnini, F., Rossi, G., Lunetta, C., Banfi, P., & Corbo, M. (2010). Clinical psychology and amyotrophic lateral sclerosis. *Frontiers in Psychology, 1*, 5. doi: 10.3389/fpsyg.2010.00033.

Pagnini, F., Simmons, Z., Corbo, M., & Molinari, E. (2012). Amyotrophic lateral sclerosis: Time for research on psychological intervention? *Amyotrophic Lateral Sclerosis*. doi: 10.3109/17482968.2011.653572.

Rabkin, J. G., Wagner, G. J., & Del Bene, M. (2000). Resilience and distress among amyotrophic lateral sclerosis patients and caregivers. *Psychosomatic Medicine, 62*(2), 271-279.

Simmons, Z. (2005). Management strategies for patients with amyotrophic lateral sclerosis from diagnosis through death. *Neurologist, 11*(5), 257-270. doi: 00127893-200509000-00001 [pii]

Simmons, Z., Felgoise, S. H., Bremer, B. A., Walsh, S. M., Hufford, D. J., Bromberg, M. B., et al. (2006). The ALSSQOL: balancing physical and nonphysical factors in assessing quality of life in ALS. *Neurology, 67*(9), 1659-1664. doi: 67/9/1659 [pii] 10.1212/01.wnl.0000242887.79115.19.

Talbot, K. (2002). Motor neurone disease. *Postgraduate Medical Journal, 78*(923), 513-519.

Thoresen, C. E. (1998). Spirituality, health and science: the coming revival? In S. Roth-Roemer, S. E. Robinson-Kurpius & C. Carmin (Eds.), *The Emerging Role of Counseling Psychology in Health Care*. New York: Norton.

Van den Berg, J. P., Kalmijn, S., Lindeman, E., Veldink, J. H., de Visser, M., Van der Graaff, M. M., et al. (2005). Multidisciplinary ALS care improves quality of life in patients with ALS. *Neurology, 65*(8), 1264-1267. doi: 65/8/1264 [pii] 10.1212/01.wnl.0000180717.29273.12.

Wolpe, J. (1990). *The Practice of Behavior Therapy*. Tarrytown, NY: Pergamon Press.

Worms, P. M. (2001). The epidemiology of motor neuron diseases: a review of recent studies. *Journal of the Neurological Sciences, 191*(1-2), 3-9. doi: S0022510X0100630X [pii].

In: Amyotrophic Lateral Sclerosis
Editors: Katashi Segawa and Ryota Ijichi
ISBN: 978-1-62257-679-1

Chapter 6

Amyotrophic Lateral Sclerosis and Lipid Peroxidation

***Moses Henderson*[1], *Seth Van Zant*[1] *and Tanea T. Reed*[1,*]**
[1] Department of Chemistry, Eastern Kentucky University, Richmond, KY, US

Abstract

Amyotrophic lateral sclerosis (ALS) is a neurodegenerative disorder that affects 1 in 50,000 persons. Symptoms begin to develop between 40 and 70 years old, but can occur as young as 30 years of age [5]. Also known as Lou Gehrig's disease, ALS patients demonstrate twitching and overall muscle weakness. Eventually, the disease spreads to other areas of the body, causing muscle atrophy marked by motor neuron degeneration in the central nervous system leading to loss of voluntary muscle control. Amyotrophic lateral sclerosis is a fatal disorder which typically leads to death within three to five years after initial onset of symptoms. Although the majority of ALS cases are sporadic, the exact cause is unknown. Furthermore, only 5-10% of all ALS cases are classified as familial. Current literature bolsters a mutation in the antioxidant enzyme, superoxide dismutase 1 (SOD1), as a possible causative agent, yet only 10% of all ALS patients have this specific genetic mutation [5]. The SOD1 mutation reduces the ability to reduce harmful free radicals, thereby promoting lipid peroxidation and inducing higher levels of lipid peroxidation end products (i.e. acrolein, 4-hydroxy-2-nonenal, malondialdehyde). Lipid peroxidation is a multifaceted biochemical process involving the interaction of polyunsaturated fatty acids with oxygen- containing free radicals in turn generating a plethora of highly reactive electrophilic aldehydes. This article will focus on the relationship between amyotrophic lateral sclerosis and lipid peroxidation, specifically the current pharmacological treatments associated with the alteration of lipid metabolism to treat the symptoms of this debilitating disease.

Keywords: Amyotrophic lateral sclerosis, lipid peroxidation, superoxide dismutase, lipid metabolism

* Address correspondence and reprint requests to: Professor Tanea T. Reed, Department of Chemistry, Eastern Kentucky University, Richmond, KY 40475, USA. Ph: +1-859-622-1459; Fax: +1-859-622-8197; E-mail: tanea.reed@eku.edu.

INTRODUCTION

Amyotrophic Lateral Sclerosis (ALS) is a neurodegenerative disease that affects both the upper and lower motor neurons. Until recently, research was sparse on this motor disorder. It was not until 1939, when Lou Gehrig was diagnosed, that the general public became more aware of this disease and large scale research efforts began. Gehrig began his prolific baseball career in 1923 with the New York Yankees and played a record setting 2,130 consecutive games. In 1938, Gehrig's batting average slipped, and he began noticing that his strength was fading. In 1939, just eight games into the season, Gehrig pulled himself from the starting lineup. Later that season, doctors at the Mayo Clinic diagnosed Gehrig with amyotrophic lateral sclerosis, thereby ending his career.

ALS affects both upper (brain) and lower (spinal and bulbar innervating) motor neurons. These motor neurons serve as communication pathways between the brain and the voluntary muscles of the body. The gradual degeneration and death of motor neurons has devastating effects throughout the body. As degeneration continues, the neurons are inhibited and the brain begins to lose functional control of these muscles, until progressive atrophy renders them useless. While ALS has an incidence rate of only 1-2 in 50,000, it is not considered a rare disease [2]. ALS is one of the most common neurodegenerative diseases in the world, affecting individuals of all racial and ethnic backgrounds. Today, individuals have a 0.14 - 0.25% risk of developing ALS within their lifetime. In the United States alone, 20,000 - 30,000 individuals have been diagnosed, and another 5,000 Americans are diagnosed each year [13]. Post diagnosis, most individuals have a life expectancy of three to five years. During this timeframe, muscle strength and control greatly declines, ultimately leading to death. The majority of ALS related deaths stem from respiratory failure associated with loss of function in respiratory muscles [19].

The diagnosis of ALS is an arduous process. Initial symptoms are often overlooked. Once symptoms begin to present, physicians run a variety of diagnostic tests to ensure that these symptoms are not a result of another condition. A number of other neurodegenerative diseases and conditions can mimic or cause ALS-like symptoms. These tests help eliminate the possibility of misdiagnosis. It is important that other diseases and conditions are not confused for ALS. Patients suffering from other neurodegenerative disorders could possibly receive beneficial treatment that could greatly add to their longevity and quality of life.

ALS is a rapidly progressive disease, regardless of where it originally manifests itself or the severity of symptoms. The disease quickly spreads throughout the body; affecting all major voluntary muscle groups, gradually weakening them until they are no longer functional. Upper motor neurons generally exhibit muscle stiffness and tightness, along with exaggerated reflexes. Lower motor neurons, those of the spinal cord and voluntary muscles, show symptoms such as muscle weakness, atrophy, cramping and increased twitching and spasticity. For many patients, the first noticeable symptom is trouble swallowing (dysphagia), due to the decreased function of muscles in the throat and mouth. As symptoms progress, patients will lose the ability to perform basic functions using their arms and legs, due to loss of movement. Eventually, the disease will advance to the point where the muscles of the respiratory system begin to be impacted. At this point, breathing complications become one of the main concerns for patients. Patients rely on ventilators and other forms of artificial breathing to help maintain the necessary oxygen supply. Due to prolonged ventilation use, patients are at a much higher risk of developing pneumonia. Respiratory muscle depletion is the ultimate cause of death in most ALS cases.

There are two main categories of ALS: familial and sporadic. Familial ALS (fALS) is a genetic condition in which the disease is inherited from the previous generation. fALS cases comprise only 5-10% of all diagnosed ALS cases [19]. Most fALS cases are inherited through autosomal dominance, but cases have been reported in which they were inherited through autosomal recessive and X-linked processes [19]. To date, at least 13 forms of fALS have been identified, affecting 6 different genes [2]. Sporadic ALS (sALS) occurs through genetic mutations. These mutations can be random, but it is also believed that environmental factors may also play a pivotal role in causing these mutations. sALS constitutes 90-95% of all ALS cases. However, the majority of research efforts have been focused on understanding the genetics of fALS, and their possible implications in fALS [1].

Familial ALS, while being the less dominate faction of ALS, receives the bulk of research attention. fALS cases make up only 5-10% of the total number of ALS cases. Of those, 20% of fALS cases are linked to genetic mutations in the antioxidant enzyme, superoxide dismutase (SOD1), which is responsible for superoxide anion to hydrogen peroxide and reducing hydrogen peroxide and oxygen [23] as shown in Figure 1.

$$O_2^{\bullet -} + 2H^+ \xrightarrow{\text{SOD}} H_2O_2 + O_2$$

Figure 1. Chemical reaction involving superoxide dismutase.

Over 150 different SOD1 linked mutations have been reported. Among those mutations, two of the most common mutation types involve the gain of cytotoxic function and C-terminal truncations [26]. The degenerative effects of SOD1 linked mutations can demonstrated in a variety of different pathological pathways, including alterations in DNA and RNA metabolism, mitochondria, neurofilaments and axonal transport systems and cell organelle functions, activation and dysfunction of glial cells, elevated extracellular levels of glutamate and other excitotoxic pathways. Each of these different stressors contributes to neuronal damage and cell death [1]. However, there are a number of other gene mutations that can also lead to the development of familial ALS.

Familial ALS can also come through inherited mutations in other genes. Specific mutations have been recorded in a number of other genes, including ALS2, SETX, VAPB, ANG and TARDBP. ALS2, a specific juvenile form, affects the ALS2 gene, causing it to produce mutant forms of the protein alsin. While the exact function of alsin in the body is unknown, mutations in the DNA coding for the protein have been linked to the development of inherited ALS. Mutant forms of alsin contribute to the degenerative effects associated with ALS. ALS4 is another type of juvenile ALS. The SETX gene is also affected, causing mutation in the senataxin protein. Senataxin mutations cause alterations in RNA processing. ALS8 causes mutations in vesicle-membrane associated membrane and synaptobrevin-associated membrane protein B. These mutations affect proteins that are thought to regulate vesicle transport. Genetic mutations that cause the production of mutated vesicle transport proteins disrupt the movement of cellular content. These mutant proteins do not function properly, and cellular material, such as glutamate, is not properly transported from the cell. ALS10 affects the TARDBP gene. TARDBP codes for the TDP-43 protein, which plays an important role in transcriptional regulation [1]. With mutations in the DNA of the TARDBP gene, mutated forms of TDP-43 are produced, leading to the development of ALS10. While each of these genes affect very different processes, they all lead to the development of ALS.

Sporadic ALS comprises 90-95% of all ALS cases. While little remains known about how these cases develop, important strides have been made recently. Associations have been made between sALS cases and identified genes seen in fALS cases. Specifically, mutations in SOD1 and TARDBP genes have been seen in a number of sALS patients [1]. This new information has led researchers to believe that ALS can be acquired through heritable and random means. While genetics is a clear factor in familial cases, complex mutations and unknown environmental factors appear to be the cause of sporadic cases.

ALS and Lipid Peroxidation

Oxidative damage is suspected to play a large role in the pathogenesis of ALS, as well as many other neurodegenerative diseases. During oxidative stress, there is a drastic imbalance between radical species and antioxidants. The excess reactive species interact with essential macromolecules in the body, specifically DNA, proteins, and lipids. The modified lipids and proteins can have a devastating effect within the body. Modified proteins become less efficient, making them less functional. Lipid modifications also decrease the efficiency of the lipid's primary function. In many cases, lipids, which are key components of the cellular membrane, undergo modifications, weakening the cell membrane and leaving the cell susceptible.

Polyunsaturated fatty acids are often the most common lipid to undergo lipid peroxidation. In the brain, this is of particular importance due to low concentration levels of oxygen in the brain and the amount of readily available polyunsaturated fatty acids present [22]. Lipid peroxidation produces various highly reactive aldehydes, such as acrolein and 4-hydroxynonenal (Figures 2 and 3, respectively), through complex interactions between free radicals and polyunsaturated fatty acids. These interactions usually run along a chain of free radical reactions, producing radicals and modified lipids until terminated by a "chain breaking" molecule [17] . Chain breaking molecules are usually antioxidants, like Vitamins C and E and glutathione, or they can be free radicals that react together, forming a neutral product [17].

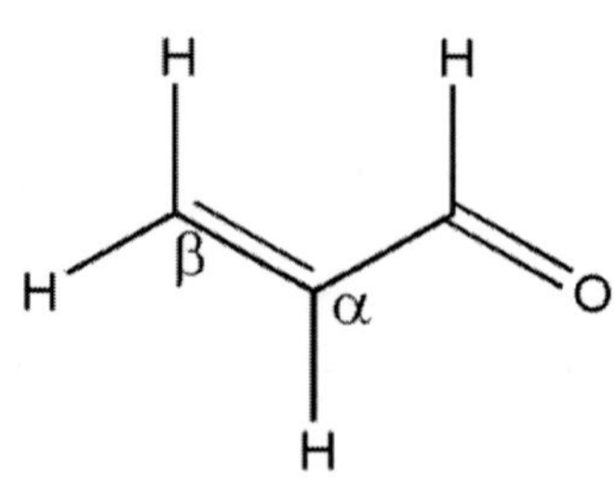

Figure 2. Structure for acrolein.

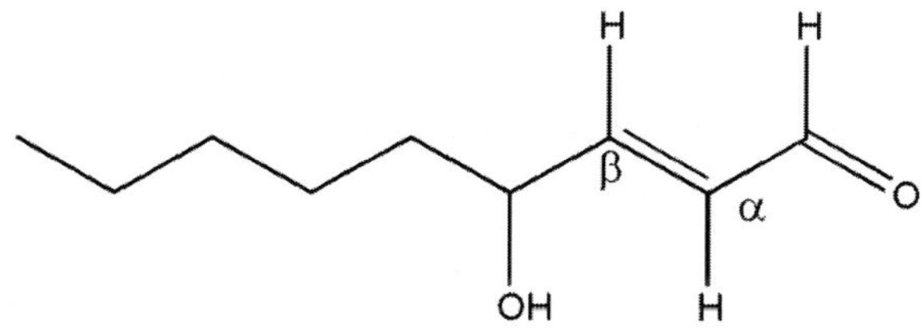

Figure 3. Structure for 4-hydroxynonenal, HNE.

Lipid peroxidation has been shown to be greatly elevated in a variety of different neurodegenerative diseases. However, it was not until the late 1990s that researchers were able to form direct links to lipid peroxidation and neurodegenerative disorders including Alzheimer's disease, Parkinson's disease, amyotrophic lateral sclerosis and Huntington's disease [11,15,16]. Thanks to the research efforts of investigators, specific biomarkers have been identified, and screening procedures are now in place. Through the screening and early detection of lipid peroxidation, diagnosis and early treatment of some neurodegenerative diseases is now possible.

Individuals suffering from amyotrophic lateral sclerosis (ALS) have been found to have increased levels of lipid peroxidation. Many cases of ALS have been linked to mutations in the zinc-copper superoxide dismutase (SOD1) gene. Mutations affecting the SOD1 protein alter its ability to efficiently and effectively harvest free radicals. It has been suspected that toxicity is a result of the misfolding of the SOD1 protein. The misfolded protein has acquired a toxic function; it has been proposed that this toxicity arises from either the catalysis of the nitrated tyrosines, or through the overproduction of hydroxyl radicals [4]. Regardless of how the toxic mutation is obtained its role in the overproduction of reactive oxygen and nitrogen species, along with its decreased function in harvesting free radicals, mutations in the SOD1 protein have been linked to increased levels of lipid peroxidation and neurodegenerative diseases. Today, researchers have been able to identify biomarkers that have direct connections to the presence of lipid peroxidation. Patients suffering from neurodegenerative diseases, specifically ALS, have been found to have abnormally high levels of these biomarkers in their sera [21].

One specific biomarker for neurodegenerative diseases is 4-hydroxy-2-nonenal (Figure 3). HNE is produced through lipid oxidation, and has been identified as a major product of lipid peroxidation that is present in increased amounts in various neurodegenerative diseases. In the SOD1 mutation, G93A-SOD1, three specific HNE protein adducts have been identified. These adducts are formed through the addition of HNE to specific amino acid residues. These modifications are toxic, causing the amino acids to lose function, and alter their role in protein production [17]. High HNE concentrations have been found to produce a number of harmful effects in vivo. Specifically, HNE has been linked to disruptions in calcium homeostasis, impairment in glutamate transportation, membrane damage and even cell death [9].

3-Nitrotyrosine (3-NT) is another prominent biomarker that has been indicated in neurodegenerative diseases. It has been identified as a "fingerprint" of reactive nitrogen species formation [3]. While many studies have recorded that 3-NT is indeed a biomarker for the production of nitrogen species, as well as oxidative stress, new research suggests that it also plays a role in cell toxicity. Nitrotyrosine is capable of acting as a neurotoxin through the inhibition, and eventual loss, of dopamanergic neurons [12]. Through prolonged exposure to 3-NT (Figure 4), dopamanergic neurons are lost through apoptotic cell death. While the pathological pathway is unclear, it is certain that 3-NT is responsible for the loss of these motor neurons [3]. These findings have shed new light on the exact role of nitrotyrosine in neurodegenerative diseases. New linkages between 3-NT and its effect on motor neurons could also help researchers in understanding what part toxic lipid metabolites play in ALS.

Acrolein (Figure 2) has also been indicated as a major contributor in the pathogenesis of neurodegeneration. When incubated, acrolein is capable of producing conjugates, joining with lysine, in various proteins and lipids [10]. Acrolein has endogenous, as well as many environmental points of origin. *In vivo*, acrolein is produced through the oxidation of polyunsaturated fatty acids. However, it can also be found in the environment through the incomplete combustion of plastics, cigarette smoke and the overheating or burning of food products [25]. Acrolein has been linked to neurodegenerative disease through its role in neurofilament aggregation. In the presence of high concentrations of acrolein, neurofilament-L (NF-L) is excessively modified. These modifications allow for the aggregation of NF-L. These aggregates resemble amyloid plaques seen in Alzheimer's disease, and have also been closely related to oxidative reactions [10]. For these two reasons, NF-L aggregates, caused by acrolein, have been linked to neurodegenerative diseases.

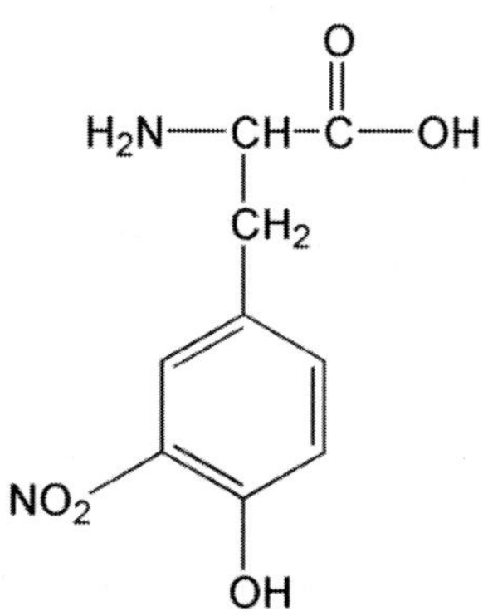

Figure 4. Structure of 3-nitrotyrosine.

Recent work has shown that acrolein, and NF-L aggregation can also lead to ALS-like symptoms. In transgenic mice studies, researchers found that overexpression of NF-L and NF aggregation can cause direct abnormalities and degeneration of motor neurons [25]. NF-L and NF aggregation has been found to be increased through acrolein, and its ability to produce free radicals [10]. These findings further support the role of lipid peroxidation in the over production of free radicals and oxidative stress as factors in neurodegenerative diseases, like ALS.

The pathogenesis of amyotrophic lateral sclerosis is still largely unexplained. However, a combination of factors, including excitotoxicity, oxidative stress and the apoptosis of motor neurons have all been suspected to contribute to its deteriorating effects [20] . Lipid peroxidation produces a number of important biomarkers that have been identified in neurodegenerative diseases. While the exact role of many of these substances is not fully understood, their presence, and the level at which they are present, in those suffering from ALS, and other neurodegenerative disorders, have made them the topic of a great deal of research. These biomarkers are now being used as targets in screening methods to help diagnose and treat patients. In the future, researchers will work to better understand the role of these molecules, as well as develop therapeutic treatments that may be able to mediate their levels, and reverse the devastating effects of the pathways that produce them.

Pharmacological Treatments

Amyotrophic lateral sclerosis is a relatively rare neurodegenerative disorder characterized by gradual decline in cognition and behavior affecting both upper and lower motor neurons. The disease of "lost memories" has become one of the most cataclysmic medical problems of the 21st century. The progression of the disease is usually rapid, ultimately leading to death within years of being diagnosed. Since there is no reversing the course of amyotrophic lateral sclerosis, the regulation of ALS is fundamentally symptom based and mainly involves deterring the progression of symptoms.

Although current available pharmacological agents, acetylcholinesterase (AChE) inhibitors and NMDA inhibitors, do not cease the development of ALS, they do provide stabilization to the classic symptoms. Both AChE and NMDA inhibitors are intended to improve cognitive aptitude, delay continual cognitive decline, and enhance the quality of life and independence as long as possible.

The most common course of treatment for individuals suffering from ALS is the use of riluzole. Riluzole, an antiglutamatinergic agent, is the only compound that demonstrated a beneficial effect on ALS patients, but with only modest increase in life expectancy. Riluzole inhibits the presynaptic release of glutamate, a chemical messenger in the brain that is often present in greater levels in people with ALS [14]. Riluzole blocks the neurotransmission in the CNS, as well as postsynaptic effects of glutamic acid (Figure 5), by noncompetitive blockade of N-methyl-D-aspartate (NMDA) (Figure 6) receptors [6].

NMDA receptors, one form of glutamate receptors, play a key role in memory and synaptic plasticity. Riluzole also contributes to the inactivation of voltage-dependent sodium channels and interferes with intracellular events that follow transmitter binding at excitatory amino acid receptors [6]. It is also believed that riluzole may improve patients' ability to swallow, as well as delay the need for ventilator assistance. At best, it is a very modest remedy for such a lethal condition [14]. Although riluzole is not a cure for ALS, it is the first and only medication approved by the Food and Drug Administration for inhibiting this disorder.

In addition to riluzole, a variety of different palliative care techniques can be used to improve the quality of life for those suffering from ALS. Medications can be prescribed to help cope with the pain and fatigue associated with the condition. In addition, other optional therapies can also provide relief. Patients can work with physical therapists to strengthen their muscles and improve their cardiovascular strength. Occupational and speech therapists can also assist those with ALS. As the disease progresses and respiratory muscles are significantly weakened, ventilators are often used to assist with breathing. Although there is no cure for ALS, the current treatment strategies can increase longevity, as well as allow patients to experience a better quality of life.

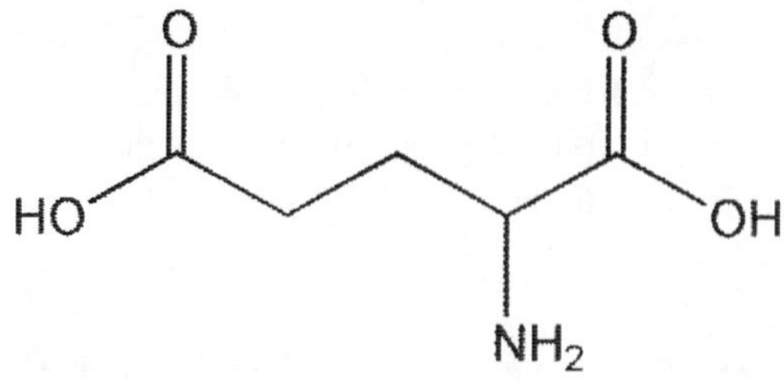

Figure 5. Structure of glutamic acid.

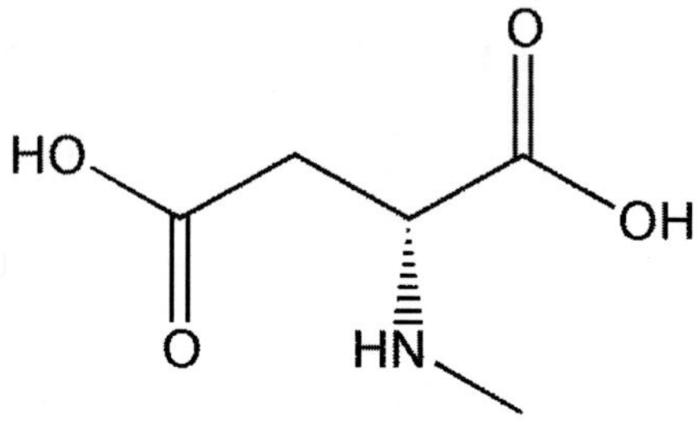

Figure 6. Structure of N-Methyl-D-aspartate (NMDA).

Of the currently approved ACE inhibitors, three are still frequently prescribed: Aricept (donepezil), Exelon (rivastigmine), and Razadyne (galantamine). Notably, all three are used to treat various stages of Alzheimer's disease, another neurrodegenerative disorder. As acetylcholine esterase inhibitors, these drugs prevent the breakdown of the neurotransmitter, acetylcholine thereby increasing its levels. Acetylcholine is essential in maintaining synaptic transmission between neurons and establishing muscle coordination, which is severely reduced in ALS patients.

Drugs such as baclofen, benzodiazepines (such as diazepam), and Elavil (amitriptyline) are also used in alleviating symptoms associated with ALS. Both baclofen and benzodiazepines are used to control unusual muscle tightness that interferes with daily movement and activities. Spasticity is caused by damage to upper motor neurons and to the part of the brain that is involved in movements under one's own control [18]. Patients with ALS also exhibit symptoms associated with dysarthria and dysphagia, which is the impairment of speech due to the weakness of surrounding mouth muscles resulting in excessive saliva pooling due to the inability to swallow saliva. Amitriptyline is used in patients with problems of swallowing their own saliva to prevent choking [8]. In certain cases, patients with ALS are prescribed other classes of pharmacological agents, such as antianxiety drugs, antipsychotics, and antidepressants to combat symptoms. These agents are used in patients who are exhibiting behavioral symptoms, such as depression, hallucinations, or sleep disturbances.

Deregulated lipid metabolism is of extreme importance for CNS injuries and disorders, as the brain has the largest lipid concentration next to adipose tissue [24]. Lipids are the major source of energy storage and play an intricate role in providing energy to the body. The crucial role of lipids in tissue physiology and cell signaling is validated by the many neurodegenerative diseases that involve a derestricted lipid metabolism. Two thirds of patients diagnosed with ALS develop a hypermetabolism of an unknown cause, leading to increased resting energy expenditure [7]. The relationship in ALS patients with increased metabolism, along with general lipid degeneration, complexes the nature of ALS. Hyperlipidemia, or elevated levels of lipids in the blood, was found to be more frequent by twofold in patients with ALS [7]. Increased lipid content in diets is considered a predictive factor for survival in ALS patients and aids in neuroprotection and extended survival. Lipids, specifically cholesterol, contribute heavily in the synthesis of neurosteroids which provide neuroprotective properties and can prolong survival by more than 12 months when concentrations are elevated. Lowering the levels of neurosteroids will accelerate the rate of neurotoxicity due to the lack of protection. The importance of nutritional intervention identifies the significance when treating ailing patients with specific lipid-lowering drugs.

Conclusion

Amyotrophic lateral sclerosis is a neurodegenerative disorder in which patients demonstrate twitching and overall muscle weakness. Eventually, the disease spreads to other areas of the body, causing muscle atrophy marked by motor neuron degeneration in the central nervous system leading to loss of voluntary muscle control. Amyotrophic lateral sclerosis is a fatal disorder which typically leads to death within three to five years after initial onset of symptoms. Although the majority of ALS cases are sporadic, the exact cause is unknown. Several genetic mutations in SOD1 contribute to the increased levels of lipid peroxidation demonstrated in this neurodegenerative disorder. Currently, there is no cure for this disease; however there are several therapeutic strategies that are used to treat the symptoms. Continued research efforts will further provide insight into the role of lipid peroxidation and ALS as well as new pharmacological treatments associated with the alteration of lipid metabolism to treat the symptoms of this debilitating disease.

References

[1] Beleza-Meireles, A., & Al-Chalabi, A. (2009). Genetic studies of amyotrophic lateral sclerosis: controversies and perspectives. *Amyotroph Lateral Scler, 10*(1), 1-14.

[2] Bento-Abreu, A., Van Damme, P., Van Den Bosch, L., et al. (2010). The neurobiology of amyotrophic lateral sclerosis. *Eur J Neurosci, 31*(12), 2247-2265.

[3] Blanchard-Fillion, B., Prou, D., Polydoro, M., et al. (2006). Metabolism of 3-nitrotyrosine induces apoptotic death in dopaminergic cells. *J Neurosci, 26*(23), 6124-6130.

[4] Bruijn, L. I., Beal, M. F., Becher, M. W., et al. (1997). Elevated free nitrotyrosine levels, but not protein-bound nitrotyrosine or hydroxyl radicals, throughout amyotrophic lateral sclerosis (ALS)-like disease implicate tyrosine nitration as an aberrant in vivo property of one familial ALS-linked superoxide dismutase 1 mutant. *Proc Natl Acad Sci U S A, 94*(14), 7606-7611.

[5] Costa, J., Gomes, C., & de Carvalho, M. (2010). Diagnosis, pathogenesis and therapeutic targets in amyotrophic lateral sclerosis. *CNS Neurol Disord Drug Targets, 9*(6), 764-778.

[6] Doble, A. (1996). The pharmacology and mechanism of action of riluzole. *Neurology, 47*(6 Suppl 4), S233-241.

[7] Dupuis, L., Corcia, P., Fergani, A., et al. (2008). Dyslipidemia is a protective factor in amyotrophic lateral sclerosis. *Neurology, 70*(13), 1004-1009.

[8] Engel, P. A. (1996). Treatment of progressive supranuclear palsy with amitriptyline: therapeutic and toxic effects. *J Am Geriatr Soc, 44*(9), 1072-1074.

[9] Esterbauer, H., Schaur, R. J., & Zollner, H. (1991). Chemistry and biochemistry of 4-hydroxynonenal, malonaldehyde and related aldehydes. *Free Radic Biol Med, 11*(1), 81-128.

[10] Jeong, M. S., & Kang, J. H. (2008). Acrolein, the toxic endogenous aldehyde, induces neurofilament-L aggregation. *BMB Rep, 41*(9), 635-639.

[11] Mattson, M. P. (2009). Roles of the lipid peroxidation product 4-hydroxynonenal in obesity, the metabolic syndrome, and associated vascular and neurodegenerative disorders. *Exp Gerontol, 44*(10), 625-633.

[12] Mihm, M. J., Schanbacher, B. L., Wallace, B. L., et al. (2001). Free 3-nitrotyrosine causes striatal neurodegeneration in vivo. *J Neurosci, 21*(11), RC149.

[13] Miller, R. G., Anderson, F., Brooks, B. R., et al. (2009). Outcomes research in amyotrophic lateral sclerosis: lessons learned from the amyotrophic lateral sclerosis clinical assessment, research, and education database. *Ann Neurol, 65 Suppl 1*, S24-28.

[14] Miller, R. G., Mitchell, J. D., Lyon, M., et al. (2003). Riluzole for amyotrophic lateral sclerosis (ALS)/motor neuron disease (MND). *Amyotroph Lateral Scler Other Motor Neuron Disord, 4*(3), 191-206.

[15] Montine, K. S., Quinn, J. F., Zhang, J., et al. (2004). Isoprostanes and related products of lipid peroxidation in neurodegenerative diseases. *Chem Phys Lipids, 128*(1-2), 117-124.

[16] Ou, J. J., Zhang, Y., & Montine, T. J. (2002). In vivo assessment of lipid peroxidation products associated with age-related neurodegenerative diseases. *Exp Neurol, 175*(2), 363-369.

[17] Reed, T. T. (2011). Lipid peroxidation and neurodegenerative disease. *Free Radic Biol Med, 51*(7), 1302-1319.

[18] Schinwelski, M., & Slawek, J. (2010). Prevalence of spasticity following stroke and its impact on quality of life with emphasis on disability in activities of daily living. Systematic review. *Neurol Neurochir Pol, 44*(4), 404-411.

[19] Shoichet, S. A., Waibel, S., Endruhn, S., et al. (2009). Identification of candidate genes for sporadic amyotrophic lateral sclerosis by array comparative genomic hybridization. *Amyotroph Lateral Scler, 10*(3), 162-169.

[20] Siciliano, G., D'Avino, C., Del Corona, A., et al. (2002). Impaired oxidative metabolism and lipid peroxidation in exercising muscle from ALS patients. *Amyotroph Lateral Scler Other Motor Neuron Disord, 3*(2), 57-62.

[21] Simpson, E. P., Henry, Y. K., Henkel, J. S., et al. (2004). Increased lipid peroxidation in sera of ALS patients: a potential biomarker of disease burden. *Neurology, 62*(10), 1758-1765.

[22] Subczynski, W. K., & Hyde, J. S. (1983). Concentration of oxygen in lipid bilayers using a spin-label method. *Biophys J, 41*(3), 283-286.

[23] Valdmanis, P. N., Belzil, V. V., Lee, J., et al. (2009). A mutation that creates a pseudoexon in SOD1 causes familial ALS. *Ann Hum Genet, 73*(Pt 6), 652-657.

[24] Walkley, S. U., & Suzuki, K. (2004). Consequences of NPC1 and NPC2 loss of function in mammalian neurons. *Biochim Biophys Acta, 1685*(1-3), 48-62.

[25] Xu, Z., Cork, L. C., Griffin, J. W., et al. (1993). Increased expression of neurofilament subunit NF-L produces morphological alterations that resemble the pathology of human motor neuron disease. *Cell, 73*(1), 23-33.

[26] Zetterstrom, P., Andersen, P. M., Brannstrom, T., et al. (2011). Misfolded superoxide dismutase-1 in CSF from amyotrophic lateral sclerosis patients. *J Neurochem, 117*(1), 91-99.

In: Amyotrophic Lateral Sclerosis
Editors: Katashi Segawa and Ryota Ijichi

ISBN: 978-1-62257-679-1

Chapter 7

The Spread Pattern and Survival in Sporadic ALS: "How Does ALS Progress or Propagate?"

Fumiharu Kimura*
Division of Neurology, The First Department of Internal Medicine, Osaka Medical College, Takatsukishi, Osaka, Japan

ABSTRACT

Objective: The rostral-caudal distributions of lower motor neuron (LMN) in the pontomedullary, cervical and lumbosacral segments of the CNS are related to bulbar, upper limb and lower limb symptoms, respectively.

Respiratory function will be linked to multiple motor neuron functions such as not only thoracic segment, but pontomedullary, cervical segment. A misfolding pathology involving mutant superoxide dismutase-1 and TDP-43 causing sporadic ALS has recently been suggested to spread from the site of disease onset to neighboring areas in a prion-like manner in animal models. Our aims were to clarify onset type in association with 5 year survival, the relationships between interval or sites from first symptoms to second symptoms and prognosis. We also examined the pattern of spread and direction of clinical LMN involvement over time from onset until the appearance of respiratory symptoms, and sites and frequency of normally preserved motor function at the appearance of respiratory symptoms.

Method: 150 patients with sporadic amyotrophic lateral sclerosis (ALS) underwent follow-up at 3 month intervals until the appearance of respiratory symptoms. Symptom appearances were determined using the revised version of the ALS Functional Rating Scale.

Result: Median survival with combined type onset (two regions simultaneously) was shorter (18 months) than with bulbar onset (26 months, p1/40.01). The interval from

*in1110@poh.osaka-med.ac.jp.

onset to involvement of the second region correlated significantly with survival, independent of particular combinations. Five year survival rate was 21% for lower limb onset, 18% for upper limb onset and 16% for bulbar onset. No patient with a rapid spread pattern (two regions within 3 months from onset) survived >5 years. In terms of cumulative occurrence, symptoms spread longitudinally to adjacent regions. Bulbar function remained preserved in 27%, lower limb function in 10% and upper limb function in 2.7%.

Conclusion: The data supports the contiguous anatomical propagation of LMN involvement in sporadic ALS.

INTRODUCTION

Amyotrophic lateral sclerosis (ALS) is a fatal neurodegenerative disorder that affects the spinal, brainstem and cortical motoneurons, giving rise to weakness of the upper and lower limbs, bulbar palsy, and eventual respiratory failure [1].

The pattern of spread until respiratory failure in ALS varies from patient to patient. One of the important tasks in sporadic ALS research is the spread pattern in individual patients who progress at different rates. Median survival time (MST) from initial onset until death without ventilation assistance or tracheostomy ranges from 2-4 years all over the world [2-4]. About 20% of sporadic ALS patients survive over 5 years [5].

Respiratory symptoms are generally accepted to develop late in the setting of established limb and bulbar involvement. However, unexpected respiratory failure can occur in patients with normally preserved lower motor neuron (LMN) functions [6].

This review assessed the pattern of onset including combined type, 5 years survival rate, pattern of spread at each body site over time from onset to respiratory symptoms, sites and frequency of normally preserved motor function at the appearance of respiratory symptoms, the presence or timing of bulbar symptoms and survival, and the relationship between interval or sites from first symptom to second symptom (FS-SS) and survival in sporadic ALS patients.

SPINAL REGIONAL FUNCTION

The rostral-caudal distributions of four LMNs at the pontomedullary, cervical, thoracic-truncal, and lumbosacral segments are related to bulbar (B), upper limb (U), respiratory (R) and lower limb (L) symptoms, respectively [7].

Respiratory function is widely related to thoracic-truncal segment (intercostal muscle, abdominal muscle), the innervations of phrenic nerve (diaphragma), which are located in the cervical (C3-C5) region [8] and other respiration related muscle weakness (sternocleidomastoideus) (Figure 1). Assessment of these four segmental regions is internationally performed using the El Escorial criteria [9].

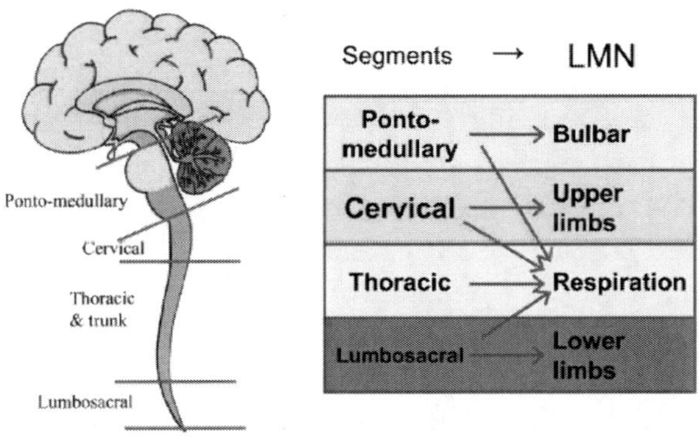

Figure 1. The rostral-caudal distributions of four lower motor neurons Respiratory function is an indispensable function to maintain life, so it is widely related to not only thoracic-truncal segment, but the cervical segment and pontomedullary segment.

PRION-LIKE PROPAGATION

A misfolding pathology involving mutant superoxide dismutase-1 (SOD1) in familial ALS and transactivation response element DNA binding protein 43 (TDP-43) associated to sporadic ALS has recently been discussed about spread from the site of disease onset to neighboring areas in a prion-like manner [10-14]. Whether this phenomenon occurs naturally in sporadic ALS remains unknown. A similar concept has been recognized in the Braak theory of Parkinson's disease regarding upward propagation from the olfactory bulb and gut autonomic nerves [15]. Analyzing the propagation of pathology from observation of LMNs phenotypes is easier in ALS than in other neurodegenerative disorders. We examined the pattern of spread or propagation and direction of clinical LMN involvement over time from onset until the appearance of respiratory symptoms.

Table 1. The association between ΔFS (at diagnosis) and the duration (from diagnosis until primary end point) in log-rank test and Cox proportional hazards models, adjusting for age at baseline and sex

	Kaplan Meier survival rate			Cox proportional Hazard model		
	N	MST	*p* (log-rank)	HR	CI	*p*
ΔFS						
group I (<0.67)	41	20.3		1		
group II (≧0.67)	41	11.5	<0.001	2.35	1.31-2.91	0.005
ΔFS						
<0.5	29	23.8		1		
0.5-1.0	28	18.4	0.021	1.96	1.11-2.33	0.019
≧1.0	25	9.23	<0.001	2.51	1.36-4.63	0.003
ALSFRS-R						
≧38	50	22.9		1		
<38	32	12.4	0.026	1.44	0.87-2.41	0.161

N, number of patients; MST, median survival time (months); HR, hazard ratio.
ΔFS = (48 - ALSFRS-R at "time of diagnosis") / Duration from onset to diagnosis (month).

ALS FUNCTIONAL RATING SCALE REVISED VERSION (ALSFRS-R)

ALSFRS-R is a 48 questionnaire-based scale using an equally weighted scale concerning four regions (U, L, B, R) [16]. It is a useful instrument to evaluate the aspects of clinical onset in each site. ALSFRS-R is sensitive to the change over time and can predict survival at diagnosis [17]. In our previous study [18], rate of progression (Δ FS) according to ALSFRS-R at the time of diagnosis predicts survival [19] (Table 1). In teams of ALSFRS-R, walking, or climbing stairs, or turning over in bed, estimated L function. U function was estimated by writing, self-feeding, or dressing, and B function was estimated by speech, salivation, or deglutition. The appearance of R was based on dyspnea at meals or while bathing, orthopnea or sleep disturbance due to dyspnea. The primary endpoint for survival was determined as a score under one or less out of 12 points in the respiratory domain on ALSFRS-R, indicating the time at which death would have occurred without tracheostomy or ventilatory assistance including full-time NIPPV. Normally preserved motor function at each site was defined as holding a full score of 12 points at the site according to the ALSFRS-R.

ONSET PATTERNS INCLUDING COMBINED TYPE

Table 2. Demographic and clinical characteristics at each phenotype of onset

	Upper limbs	Lower limbs	Bulbar	Combined	Total
N	50	52	32	16	150
Age	61.4±9.1	60.5±11.1	63.1±6.53	62.1±7.83	61.6±9.24
FS-FE	15.5±11.8	15.9±9.42	12.2±6.47	9.36±5.58	14.3±9.71
FRS-R	39.7±4.48	38.8±3.74	39.4±5.55	38.2±7.17	39.1±4.48
M/F	32/18	30/22	15/17	8/8	85/65
MST	33	32	26	18	32
P	ref	0.823	0.047	0.01	
5ys%	18	21	16	0	17
FS-SS	15.2±13.4	13.6 ±12.0	10.8±8.32	0.35 ±0.50	12.8 ±12.1
PS(person)	26(23)	24 (22)	4(4)	5 (5)	59(54)
PS %	52.0	46.2	12.5	31.3	36.0
U	0	3	1	0	4
L	9	0	3	3	15
B	17	21	0	2	40

U, L, B indicate numbers of patients in whom upper limb function was normally preserved at the onset of respiratory symptoms. FRS-D, Amyotrophic Lateral Sclerosis Functional Rating Scale revised score at diagnosis; FS-FE, interval between first symptoms and first examination; MST, median survival time; 5 year (%), percentage of patients surviving >5 years for each type of onset; PS (person), number of normally preserved sites (number of patient) at each site of onset; PS %, percentage of normally preserved sites at each site of onset; B, bulbar symptoms, ;C , combined type ;U, upper limb symptoms; L, lower limb symptoms.

ALS often starts in one part of the body, but occasionally develops in two regions simultaneously (Table 2). Combined (C) type of ALS was defined as two segmental regions presenting simultaneously at initial onset. In a total of 150 patients with sporadic ALS, onset was: U in 50 patients (33.3%); L in 52 patients (34.6%); and B in 32 patients (21.3%). Sixteen patients (10.6%) were C-type, comprising 9 patients with B and U, and 7 patients with U and L. No patients with C-type as B and L or B and R were noted. In other word, all C type of ALS patients showed an anatomical contiguous combination.

Five Years Survival Rate According to Onset Type

Patients surviving over 5 years following symptomatic onset of ALS account for 14-20% of the total ALS population [5, 20]. Patients surviving over 5 years are clinically similar in terms of age, sex, site of onset, and riluzole therapy. The frequency of 5-year survival rate has not changed over time. In our study, overall 5-year survival rate in ALS was 17%. ; 5-year survival rate was 21% for L onset, 18% for U onset, 16% for B onset and 0% for C type. Bulbar onset type is traditionally regarded as a poor survival but the proportion of 5-year survivors with bulbar onset was similar to that with limb-onset. Particularly important information from our survey was the finding that no patients with C-type ALS survived >5 years as shown in Table 2. The "rapid spread type" of ALS, presenting in two regions within 3 months from onset (=C + C [2-3]), revealed almost identical survival >5 years (Figure 2).

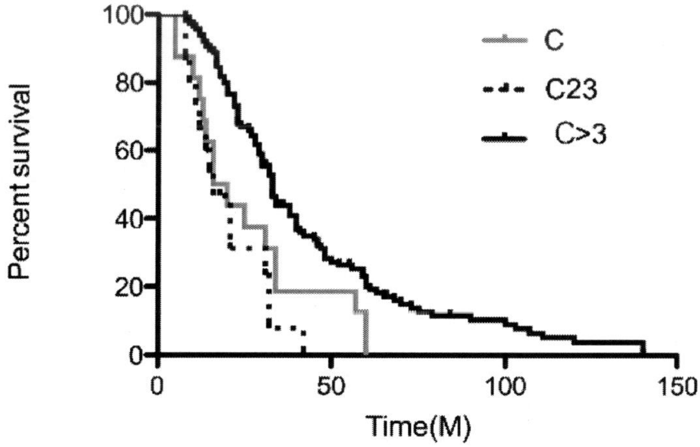

Figure 2. Kaplan Meier curves at different intervals between the first symptom and the second symptom (FS-SS).
Patients were divided into three groups: C: FS-SS within 1 month ; C2-3, FS-SS within 2-3 months. The 'rapid spread-type' of FS-SS (C+C2-3) showed significantly lower MST than other types with ALS, manifesting an FS-SS >3 M. No cases with rapid spread-type survived for more than 5 years. M, months.

SURVIVAL ACCORDING TO TIMING OF SECOND REGION

As our data displayed significantly shorter survival in C-type and rapid spread-type of ALS, we hypothesized that the interval of FS-SS offers an important predictor of survival. We confirmed that early symptom progression is related to ALS survival [21].

ALS is thought to have already undergone gradual progression by the time symptoms manifest, involving a long pre-clinical period. Progression in the early phase of ALS appears to be associated with future progression [22,23]. Cox regression analysis revealed shorter survival in patients with faster interval of FS-SS (*P*=0.002; 95% confidence interval (CI), 0.952-0.989) adjusted to age and gender.

Gowers, as far back as 1891, commented, in an entirely non-statistical way, that the early rate of progression seemed to remain consistent: "When the progress at the commencement is rapid, it usually continues rapid...when it begins slowly, it is usually slow throughout" [24]. Progression rate reflects the rate of spread and faster involvement of a second region may explain the speed of propagation in pathological aggregational mechanism.

SURVIVAL ACCORDING TO FS-SS REGIONAL COMBINATIONS

In terms of initial direction of spread, no significant difference was found between patients with L onset and B onset followed by spread to a contiguous region or skipped region and U onset spread to rostral (B) or caudal (L) site as shown in Figure 3, although no patient with B onset skipped to L survived more than 5 years.

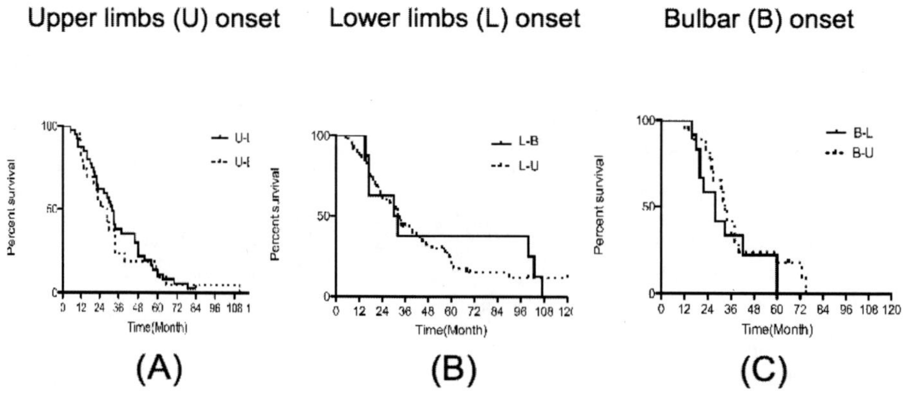

Figure 3. Kaplan Meier survival curves for combinations of first and second symptoms.
(A) group with U onset spread to L (U-L, MST: 32 M) or to B (U-B, MST 29 M)).
(B) Group with L spread to U (L-U, MST 32 months) or to B (L-B, MST 31 M).
(C) Group with B spread U (B-U, MST 28 M) or L (B-L, MST 25M). There was no significant difference in survival between contiguous spread pattern and non- contiguous spread pattern.

These findings indicated that the second-affected site did not influence survival. That is, survival was not linked to any particular combination of FS-SS, but rather to the interval of FS-SS. However, our samples were too small (From B onset to L; 12 patients, from L onset to B; 8 patients) for determining this problem. After our publication, Gargiulo-Monachelli et al reported that the type of non-contiguous spread account for the poorer prognosis than type of contiguous spread and non-contiguous spread pattern had the shortest MST [25]. The characteristics and meanings of patients with the skipping spread (multiple hits mechanism, etc) must be further examined in contrary to the usual contiguous spread patterns.

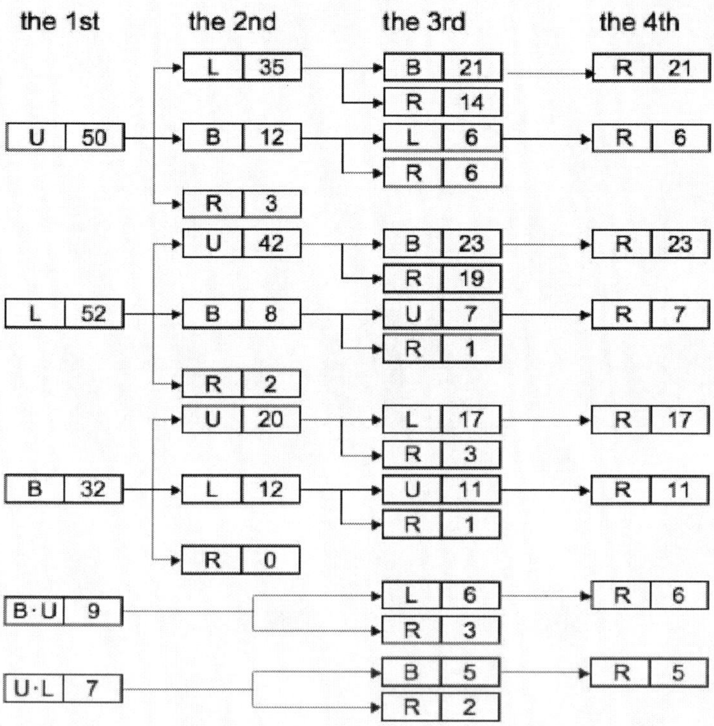

Figure 4. Patterns of spread through the order of LMN involvements from onset (1st:first symptom(s)) until respiratory symptoms.
Left side of the box shows symptom site (U, L, B, R) and the right side of the box shows numbers of patients. 'B,U' 'U,L' represents combined-type of ALS.

Motor Function Preservation at the Time of Respiratory Failure

The patterns of spread in a total of 150 sporadic ALS patients were expressed as first- (site of onset), second-, and third-order LMNs (U, L, and B) until the appearance of R. Figure 4 shows the orders of spread in the entire course from initial onset until R. R developed as the second region in 5 patients (3.3%) and as the third region in 49 patients (32.6%), as the last region in 96 patients (64%). There were approximately one-third of ALS patients who presented one or more preserved motor functions at the time of respiratory symptoms. B function was normally preserved in 40 patients (26.7%), L in 15 patients (10%), and U in 4 patients (2.7%) in Figure 5. The lowest frequency of preservation was thus seen for U, and the highest for B. Patients with L onset frequently showed preserved normal B function at the appearance of R (40.4%). One reason for the low rate (2.7%) of preservation for U function appears to be that the cervical region is anatomically located between the lumbosacral region linked to L and the pontomedullary region linked to B. As another reason, deterioration of respiratory function appears closely related to U, likely due to a link to diaphragmatic function [26,27]. The involvement of U functions appears to represent a necessary step to the development of respiratory failure.

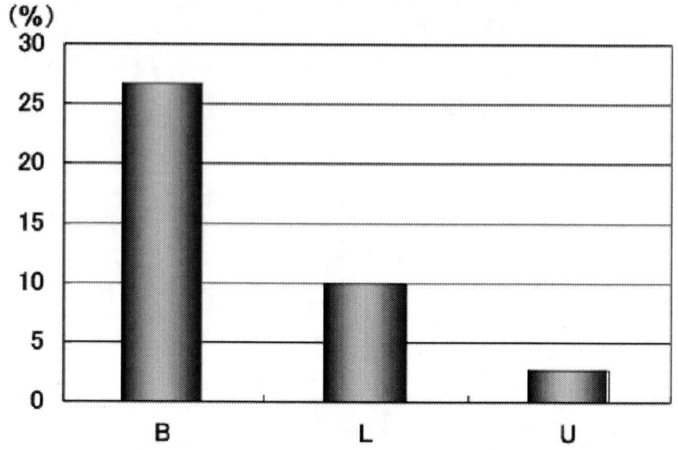

Figure 5. The frequency of normal motor sites at appearance of respiratory symptom in ALS.

SPREAD PATTERN AND SURVIVAL

When the course started with L, including C-type, 83% of cases were followed by U, 3% by R and 14% by B. When the course began with B, 71% of cases were followed by U, 29% by L and 0% by R. When the course began with U, 64% of cases were caudally followed by L, 5% by R and 32% were rostrally followed by B (Figure 4).

The development of symptoms from B onset frequently involved the anatomically close U site as compared to L. The development of symptoms from L onset also more frequently affected the nearby U than B. Anatomical non-contiguous spread of ALS was 20 patients (= 13%: 12 patients with B onset to L and 8 patients with L to B).

Cumulative occurrences of symptomatic involvement from onset to the second region are longitudinally shown in Figure 6. From the analyses of duration until occurrence in 50% of patients on Kaplan Meier plots, patients with B onset developed U (9 months) more rapidly than L (14 months, $P<0.001$, Figure 6(A)).

Patients with L onset developed U (10 months) more rapidly than B (27 months, $P<0.001$, Figure 6(B)). Patients with U onset developed faster spread to caudal (L, 14 months) than rostral (B, 17 months) regions but there was no significant difference between them ($p=0.196$, Figure 6(C)). From the analyses of cumulative occurrences, the development of LMN involvement also demonstrated anatomically contiguous spread to body regions. The analyses of cumulative occurrences revealed that L onset patients showed spread to U or rarely a skip to B. Symptoms subsequent to B onset frequently involved the anatomically close U as compared to more distant L [28].

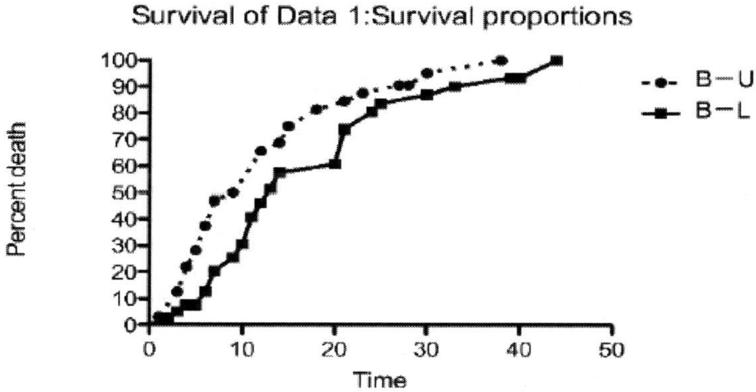

(A)

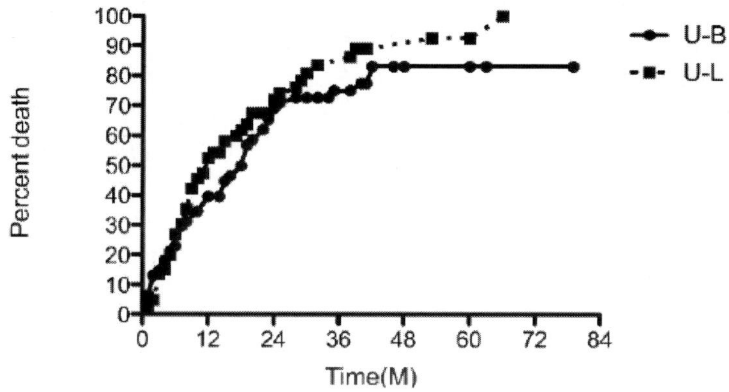

(B)

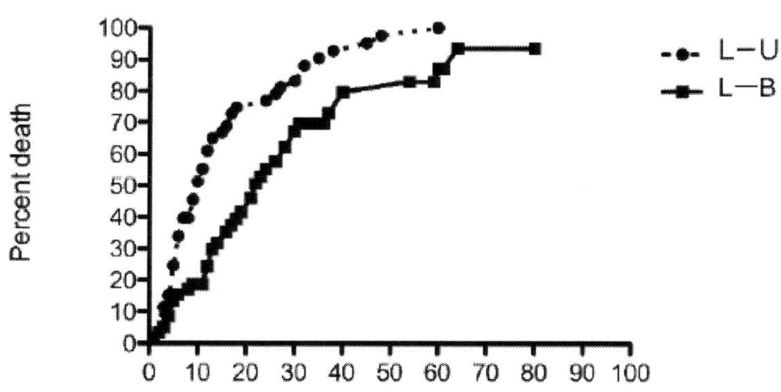

(C)

Figure 6. Cumulative occurrence of each body site in ALS.
Symptomatic involvement over time from B (A), L(B) and U (C).
Rostral spread after onset of L was faster with spread to U than with skipping spread to B, and vice versa. Occurrence of rostral (B) and caudal spread (L) was similar from U onset.

Bulbar Symptom and Prognosis

Patients were divided into two groups depending on whether they had B involvement at the time of respiratory insufficiency (Figure 7). No significant difference in survival was seen between groups with B symptoms (32 months, n=110) and spared B symptoms for the entire course (32 months, n=40, P=0.51). However, survival was significantly shorter when B symptoms developed within 12 months after initial onset (MST, 23 months, n=58) than when B symptoms developed after this time (p<0.001, n=52). Early manifestation of B symptoms within 1 year was also an important predictor of lower MST. Bulbar symptoms at diagnosis of ALS are a hallmark distinguishing this disease from other benign amyotrophic diseases, such as spinal muscle atrophy. Clinically, patients with B onset show earlier respiratory dysfunction. Bulbar symptoms directly or indirectly accompany respiratory symptoms. Directly, food, saliva or a mixture of both can enter the lung and cause aspiration pneumonia, reducing lung compliance [29, 30]. Indirectly, difficulties with communication impair quality of life [31]. Bulbar symptoms are thus thought to represent an accelerator for the development of respiratory symptoms. However, this does not present as a process connecting pontomedullary motoneuron loss to anterior horn cell loss causing respiratory dysfunction. From our survey, appearance of bulbar palsy did not reveal a positive impact on earlier respiratory dysfunction. The reason for the poor prognosis in patients with bulbar onset thus remains unclear. One possibility is that malnutrition based on bulbar symptoms promotes progression of overall muscle atrophy, with respiration-related muscle weakness influencing pulmonary function [32, 33].

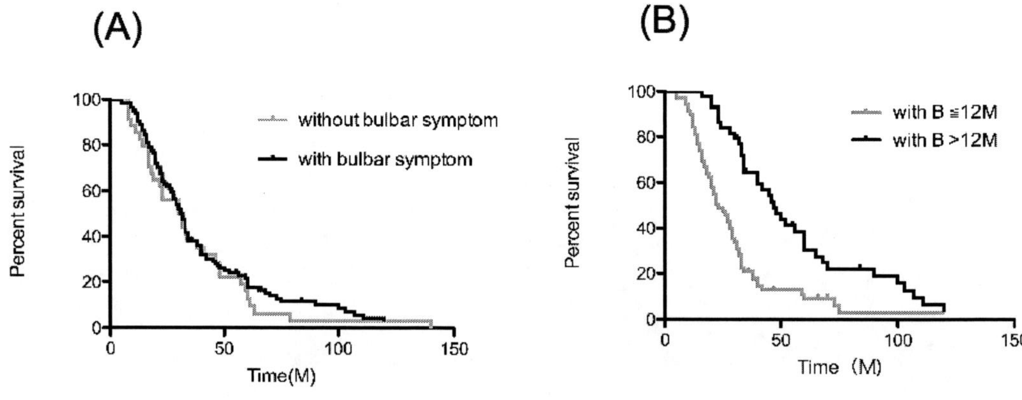

Figure 7. Kaplan Meier survival plots of ALS patients with and without bulbar symptoms. (A) ALS patient groups with B at any time in the entire course (MST 31 M) and without B symptom (MST 33 M) until respiratory symptom (B) ALS patient group displaying B within 12 months after initial onset (MST 21 M) or >12 months after initial onset (MST 47 M,).

Upper Motor Neuron (UMN) and Lower Motor Neuron (LMN)

ALS is characterized clinically and neuropatholocally by involvements of both LMN and UMN. According to the El Escorial criteria, a definite diagnosis of ALS requires both UMN and LMN involvements. The disease starts with focal process in one LMN region where both UMN and LMN are involved, but the disease progression advances separately and independently at each level [34]. No decision has been made for the question that ALS is a disease primarily of the corticomotor neuron and/or spinal motor neuron. All rating scales, including the ALSFRS-R, do not clearly differentiate between UMN and LMN impairment. For instance, gait will be impaired by UMN involvement with or without lower limb LMN involvement. Speech and swallowing dysfunctions represent a mixture of corticobulbar and bulbar involvements. The presence of LMN signs is based on physical findings including muscle atrophy and fasciculation. We did not analyze UMN signs in our survey [35] because the severity of LMN reflects the degree of UMN in addition to poor constancy of UMN signs. Another question remains as to whether the spread is first to the corticomotor neuron or spinal motor neuron. At the LMN level, spread is first to the contiguous contralateral areas and subsequent spread to the ipsilateral areas. At the UMN level, spread is first to the contiguous ipsilateral areas and subsequent spread to the contralateral areas. It is likely to spread on the spinal level because of faster involvement in contralateral site rather than rostral-caudal site.

Conclusion

Although the spread to non-contiguous regions was observed in 13% of patients, the most common direction of spread was contiguous if it spreads from U to L or B is considered to be contiguous. This finding supports the notion that the ALS pathology gradually spreads to adjacent regions in a longitudinal manner. Spread thus seems to occur in a prion-like manner without infectious ability. In most of ALS patients, the spread appears to have a contiguous pattern rather than a random pattern of progression, but not all patterns of spread were contiguous. Furthermore, time from onset to spread to the second site is a strong predictor for survival. Spread to a non-adjacent region in small numbers of patients assumed the occurrence of multi-focal hits disease progression. Although precise mechanisms of symptom spread in ALS are not understood, knowledge about the pattern of onset and the anatomical direction of spread may provide valuable prognostic insights.

This work was supported by the Osaka Medical Research Foundation for Incurable Diseases in Japan 2011.

References

[1] Haverkamp, L.J., Appel, V., Appel, S.H. Natural history of amyotrophic lateral sclerosis in a database population. Validation of a scoring system and a model for survival prediction. *Brain* 1995;118:707-719.

[2] Lee, J.R., Annegers, J.F., Appel, S.H. Prognosis of amyotrophic lateral sclerosis and the effect of referral selection. *J Neurol Sci* 1995;132:207-215.

[3] Kimura, F., Shinoda, K., Fujiwara, S., et al. The changes of clinical characteristics in 100 Japanese amyotrophic lateral sclerosis patients between 1980 and 2000 (in Japanese). *Rinsho Shinkeigaku* 2003;43:385-391.

[4] Nalini, A., Thennarasu, K., Gourie-Devi, M., et al. Clinical characteristics and survival pattern of 1, 153 patients with amyotrophic lateral sclerosis: experience over 30 years from India. *J Neurol Sci* 2008;272:60-70.
[5] Mateen, F.J., Carone, M., Sorenson, E.J. Patients who survive 5 years or more with ALS in Olmsted County, 1925-2004. *J Neurol Neurosurg Psychiatry* 2010;81:1144-1146.
[6] Kimura, F., Fujimura, C., Ishida, S., et al. A study of bulbar, upper extremity, and lower extremity motor function preservation at the time that respiratory symptoms appear in ALS (in Japanese). *Rinsho Shinkeigaku* 2007;47:140-146.
[7] Ravits, J., Paul, P., Jorg, C. Focality of upper and lower motor neuron degeneration at the clinical onset of ALS. *Neurology* 2007;68:1571-1575.
[8] Pinto, S., Geraldes, R., Vaz, N., et al. Changes of the phrenic nerve motor response in amyotrophic lateral sclerosis. longitudinal study. *Clin Neurophysiol* 2009;120:2082-2085.
[9] World Federation of Neurology Research Group on neuromuscular diseases. Subcommittee on motor neuron diseases "El Escorial World Federation of Neurology criteria for the diagnosis of amyotrophic lateral sclerosis". *J Neurol Sci* 1994;124:96-107.
[10] Münch, C., O'Brien, J., Bertolotti, A. Prion-like propagation of mutant superoxide dismutase-1 misfolding in neuronal cells. *Proc Natl Acad Sci U S A 2011*;108:3548-3553.
[11] Arai, T., Hasegawa, M., Akiyama, H., et al. TDP-43 is a component of ubiquitin-positive tau-negative inclusions in frontotemporal lobar degeneration and amyotrophic lateral sclerosis. *Biochem Biophys Res Commun* 2006;351:602-611.
[12] Hasegawa, M., Nonaka, T., Tsuji, H., et al. Molecular dissection of TDP-43 proteinopathies. *J Mol Neurosci* 2011;45:480-485.
[13] Kuwabara, S., Yokota, T. Propagation: Prion-like mechanisms can explain spreading of motor neuronal death in amyotrophic lateral sclerosis? *J Neurol Neurosurg Psychiatry* 2011;82: 1181-1182.
[14] Kanouchi, T., Ohkubo, T., Yokota, T. Can regional spreading of amyotrophic lateral sclerosis motor symptoms be explained by prion-like propagation? *J Neurol Neurosurg Psychiatry* 2012 Jul;83(7):739-745.
[15] Braak, H., Tredici, D.K. Invited article: Nervous system pathology in sporadic Parkinson disease. *Neurology* 2008;70:1916-1925.
[16] Cedarbaum, J.M., Stambler, N., Malta, E., et al. The ALSFRS-R: a revised ALS functional rating scale that incorporates assessments of respiratory function. BDNF ALS Study. *J Neurol Sci* 1999;169:13-21
[17] Kaufmann, P., Levy, G., Thompson, J.L., et al. The ALSFRSr predicts survival time in an ALS clinic population. *Neurology* 2005;64:38-43.
[18] Kimura, F., Fujimura, C., Ishida, S., et al. Progression rate of ALSFRS-R at time of diagnosis predicts survival time in ALS. *Neurology* 2006;66:265-267.
[19] Kollewe, K., Mauss, U., Krampfl, K., et al. ALSFRS-R score and its ratio: a useful predictor for ALS-progression. *J Neurol Sci* 2008;275:69-73.
[20] Wijesekera, L.C., Mathers, S., Talman, P., et al. Natural history and clinical features of the flail arm and flail leg ALS variants. *Neurology* 2009;72:1087-1094.

[21] Chio, A., Mora, G., Leone, M., et al; Piemonte and Valle d'Aosta Register for ALS (PARALS). Early symptom progression rate is related to ALS outcome: a prospective population-based study. *Neurology* 2002;59:99-103.

[22] Tysnes, O.B., Vollset, S.E., Larsen, J.P., et al. Prognostic factors and survival in amyotrophic lateral sclerosis. *Neuroepidemiology* 1994;13:226-235.

[23] Del Aguila, M.A., Longstreth, W.T. Jr., McGuire, V., et al. Prognosis in amyotrophic lateral sclerosis. A population-based study. *Neurology* 2003;60:813-19.

[24] Gowers, W.R. *Diseases of the Nervous System.* P. Blakiston, Son & Co. Philadelphia 1893:483.

[25] Gargiulo-Monachelli, G.M., Janota, F., Bettini, M., Shoesmith, C.L., Strong, M.J., Sica, R.E. Regional spread pattern predicts survival in patients with sporadic amyotrophic lateral sclerosis. *Eur J Neurol.* 2012 Jun;19(6):834-841.

[26] Similowski, T., Attali, V., Bensimon, G., et al. Diaphragmatic dysfunction and dyspnoea in amyotrophic lateral sclerosis. *Eur Respir J* 2000;15:332-337.

[27] Sathyaprabha, T.N., Pradhan, C., Nalini, A., et al. Pulmonary function tests and diaphragmatic compound muscle action potential in patients with sporadic amyotrophic lateral sclerosis. *Acta Neurol Scand* 2010;121:400-405.

[28] Brooks, B.R. Natural history of ALS: symptoms, strength, pulmonary function, and disability. *Neurology* 1996;47(Suppl 2): 71-81.

[29] Hardiman, O. Symptomatic treatment of respiratory and nutritional failure in amyotrophic lateral sclerosis. *J Neurol* 2000;247:245-251.

[30] Marin, B., Desport, J.C., Kajeu, P., et al. Alteration of nutritional status at diagnosis is a prognostic factor for survival of amyotrophic lateral sclerosis patients. *J Neurol Neurosurg Psychiatry* 2011;82:628-634.

[31] Lou, J.S., Moore, D., Gordon, P.H., et al. Correlates of quality of life in ALS: lessons from the minocycline study. *Amyotroph Lateral Scler* 2010;11:116-121.

[32] Desport, J.C., Preux, P.M., Truong, T.C., et al. Nutritional status is a prognostic factor for survival in ALS patients. *Neurology* 1999;53:1059-1063.

[33] Lou, J.S., Moore, D., Gordon, P.H., et al. Correlates of quality of life in ALS: lessons from the minocycline study. *Amyotroph Lateral Scler* 2010;11:116-121.

[34] Ravits, J., Laurie, P., Fan, Y., et al. Implications of ALS focality: rostralecaudal distribution of lower motor neuron loss postmortem. *Neurology* 2007;68:1576-1582.

[35] Fujimura-Kiyono, C., Kimura, F., Ishida, S., et al. Onset and spreading patterns of lower motor neuron involvements predict survival in sporadic amyotrophic lateral sclerosis. *J Neurol Neurosurg Psychiatry* 2011;82:1244-1249.

Index

B

C

D

E

F

G

H

N

O

P

Q

R

S

T

U

V

W

Y

Z